MW01231900

Toddler and Positive Discipline

The Ultimate Guide to Raise Respectful, Responsible and Capable Kids. Learn Effective Strategies to Develop Your Child's Abilities

By

Emma Campbell

Table of Contents

PART 1) TODDLER DISCIPLINE

PART 2) POSITIVE DISCIPLINE

PART 1

Toddler Discipline

Introduction

It is likely that you picked up this book because you are already nervous about some part of the conduct of your child and want to learn about how to best handle some of the difficult situations you are in. You are not alone and that is not uncommon for your kid. Being a parent is often challenging, fretting, and frustrating. How do you decide which course of action is best? We always feel guilty; we are unsure of how to respond; we are worried about being the cause of the issue. Often, we feel tired, unhappy, resentful, exasperated, and stressed out by the burden and everyday drudgery of caring for young children. The joy they can offer is unmatched but you can sweat out the pressure and constant demands for affection, love, and care. It is no simple becoming a mom. The joy and anticipation of a new baby's birth will easily be overshadowed with fear and confusion over how to handle his screaming, eating, and sleeping. Suddenly, this little individual has demanded that you must interpret and satisfy. For the first time, you are in control of another future. You are here

Responsible for its care, growth, and development. How do you decide what you will be doing? Is it coming naturally? Do you ask how to manage things better? Generally, all of us muddle together with a mix of advice from our family members, our relatives, our friends, articles, television, newspapers, and magazines and hope it works out. We try our utmost, we love our kids and we believe our affection will outweigh whatever errors we may create along the road. This is not a reaction book because nobody will have the correct answer to all problems. Every child is like no other human, and each family in which a baby is conceived into has its past. This book can offer you ways to talk about problems that happen with your infants so you can find the best answer for you and your family.

Chapter 1: Understanding Your Toddler's Development

What is it like being a baby? This question would have seemed absurd for centuries: there was a mostly empty head behind that adorable facade. After all, an infant lacks many of the qualities that characterize the human intellect, including vocabulary and the capacity to think. Rene Descartes claimed that the young child is tied by touch, hopelessly stuck in here and now in the overwhelming sprint. In this way, a baby is only a lump of desire, a set of reflexes, and only wants to cry or be fed. Worrying like a kid implies not worrying at all. Modern science has generally agreed, trying to spend decades outlining all the things babies were unable to do because their brains had yet to develop. They could not focus, postpone pleasure, or even communicate their wishes. The Princeton philosopher Peter Singer has famously proposed that "killing a disabled infant is not morally equal to killing a human.

Yet now psychologists have begun to radically rethink their definition of the mind of an infant. They have revealed that the baby brain is abuzz with activity by using new research techniques and tools, capable of learning incredible amounts of knowledge in a relatively short time. Unlike the adult mind, which limits itself to a small slice of reality, kids may carry on a far broader range of experiences-they are more aware of the universe than we are, in a substantial way.

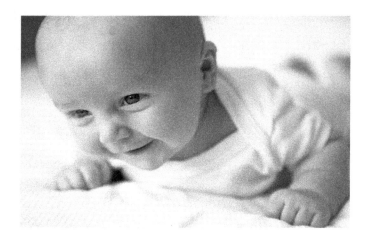

1.1 How Babies Experience the World?

It can seem like your infant does nothing but feed, sleep, scream, and fill her diapers at the very beginning. However, your child is thinking, too. She is willing to see and understand what is going on around her and express her desires and concerns to others. By interacting with her, parents will help their babies understand. Infants can see faces and objects of various shapes, sizes, and colors. They will say the difference in their parents' voices and those of others. We are shocked when we see their shapes shaped onto our limbs or legs. We are shocked by how they come into the universe capable of biting, expressing those wishes through weening and even soothing themselves. Many babies can do all these things as quickly as they are born.

In addition, this hyperawareness offers many benefits. This helps small ones, for example, to sort out their environment at a rapid speed. While babies are born entirely powerless, within a few years, they have learned everything from vocabulary to complicated motor skills such as movement-a baby learns ten new words every day. Thanks to this modern understanding of the baby brain, many of the behavioral characteristics that used to look as cognitive defects, such as the failure of children to concentrate their attention, are, in reality, essential tools in the learning cycle. In reality, in some instances, regressing into a newborn state of mind can potentially be safer for adults. Although sophistication has its benefits, it may also hinder imagination, and lead people to concentrate on the wrong information. If we need to go through tons of apparently unrelated details or construct something entirely different, our best choice is to think like an infant.

Hearing

For the first time, even before your child makes her sing to sleep, she has heard you speak to your partner and interact with your neighbor. During week 34, comfortable in your belly, your infant can feel your breathing, blood flow, and voice's soothing buzz. How do we understand exactly? Research has found that newborns favor their mothers' views to those of others; newborn babies suck at the tone of their mum's voice rather than other women's. In reality, children come to this planet hearing as much as adults do — maybe even better, because they are yet to experience their first live show on earsplitting!

Taste and Smell

Have you ever gazed into your newborn's face and wondered what is going on in her world? Could she feel the flowers growing in your garden? Is she feeling soothed by your hand touch? Is she getting excited when she listens to music? The response to each is, of course, a clear yes. Except for sight, babies arrive in the world with a reasonably well advanced majority of their senses. In reality, their sensory experiences begin long before they join the outside world of the womb. These formative experiences are far more than just practicing hearing or tasting — they are how your baby gets to know you and starts forming a strong parent-child bond. Continue reading to find out what your little one is living through in her new world.

The Nose Knows

You would be surprised to know but your baby is also an experienced sniffer at conception since the olfactory senses are developed by the time the first trimester ends. Amniotic fluid carries on the fragrance of what you consume and drink, and in utero, the child senses — and has a tolerance for — the scents of what you consume. Studies of French mothers drinking a pleasant anise-flavored soft drink during pregnancy discovered that their babies had a particular fondness for the odor of anise after birth. Whereas, for the babies whose mothers did not drink anise showed aversion or neutral reaction to the scent. Babies prefer sweet-smelling things, but they could like even preference of citrus fruit. However, it is the mother's own fragrance, which most newborns enjoy. One research showed that babies favored breast pads used by their lactating mothers over those of another lactating mother only one day after childbirth. Babies are attracted to the unadorned smell of their mother's body — so do not worry about the occasionally skipped shower. Your child will always love it.

About Taste

Your child starts developing taste buds eight weeks soon after conception. The baby's taste buds are level headed by 14 weeks, as well as she specimens all of her mother's favorite foods by ingesting amniotic fluid. She begins loving the delicious taste of frozen yogurt or flavorful pizza abundance even before she has the first sips of food or breast milk. Babies favor sweet flavors over all others at conception, a normal inclination that guarantees sensitivity to breast milk's sweet taste. As for the sense of smell, your kid would enjoy common foods — those you eat during breastfeeding, in particular. In addition, if you were eating carrot soup and baked potatoes, you could be growing a veggie lover! Babies whose mothers consumed carrot juice when breastfeeding and nursing preferred more carrot-flavored food in another analysis of baby taste tastes than children whose mothers did not.

Touch and See

Your baby can perceive a soothing touch from the beginning, differentiate a warm sensation from a cold sensation, and experience the gratification of a loving massage. Research indicates that contact will elicit strong reactions in infants;

baby stimulation is a soother surefire; and usually, premature infants who receive contact therapy accumulate weight more rapidly. In addition, do babies love feeling stuff the way they like being touched? At first, not. While newborns are as eager to reach and feel as older children, they respond to externals with their mouths and not with the hands until they hit the 4- or 5-month mark. After that, the sky is the limit — the adventurous little fingers of your baby can do anything from testing her breakfast contents to wiggling your head.

The Eyes

In comparison to the other perceptions, seeing is not well-formed in utero, despite the fact that your child can open and shut her eyes at about 32 weeks of gestation and discern between darkness and light inside the womb. Many mothers say that a spotlight shone on their abdomen triggers their kid to turn towards or away from the sun. The universe seems like a blurred, dark-and-white location to a child. She is limited to only seeing things 8 to 12 inches away when trying to feed her, really about the length to your face. Therefore, it should not be surprising to know she loves to stare at you! Babies like to gaze at the human face. Babies can better perceive high-comparison items at this point — they are particularly drawn to the shape of the face or hairline, which is easier to discern due to the contrast. Therefore, a kid can more quickly see a plush panda bear than a pastel rabbit. Of reality, an infant may not be able to see her baby quilt's varying hues yet; her capacity to see colors starts to grow about eight weeks, as forms take on more meaning. Her vision should strengthen after at least four months. Your child will acquire binocular vision, the capacity to concentrate and perceive depth in addition to seeing colors. (Before her eyes may have clashed if she could not focus well.) Mix this with her developing motor abilities, and you have a kid that is happy to play — she will grab for dolls, bright earrings, and everything else that catches her attention. After she achieves a monocular vision for around seven months, the final sensory landmark occurs the capacity to concentrate and sense distance with only one hand. The learned abilities will eventually help her manage running and walking.

Within the Toddler's Mind

Every parent who has ever observed the serious, unblinking eyes of a kid has asked, "I wonder what she thinks?" Gaining an ever-increasing glimpse into the active mind of your infant and how it functions is a fascinating aspect of infancy. The greatest reason these feelings are exposed to you is the increasing opportunity to connect. Here is a glance at some small child's thinking processes: Why is she so curious about everything? Curiosity is the key motivator for your little discoverer. A kitten does not turn on and off interest at will; it is her nature. She utilizes all her senses to seek to make sense of the world — what are stuff, what are they doing, how they function.

Curiosity is the explanation of why a 12-month-old uses her mouth and hands to discover anything within scope. Which is when an 18-month-old is pulled like a magnet towards a sandbox. That is why a 2-year-old catches the cat's ears, pours out water from the sink, attempts to burrow through your cupboards, and beheads all the flowers through your yard. She cannot help herself – for the first time at least. Nevertheless, she will know what is ideal, and what is not. Is he feeling a sense of time? A kid cannot follow one clock or read a calendar. Typically, yesterday implies something that has occurred in the past, whether it was yesterday or six months ago. Tomorrow is a word all-purpose to the future. In reality, the notion of time a child has before the second or third grade does not match that of an adult. Your child lives more in the here and now. The way he marks time is with daily routines. In addition, a 1-year-old understands there is breakfast, lunch, and dinner afterward. He knows that dinner will be in a short time, even if he has no idea how long "five minutes" or "fifteen minutes" is when he is hungry and sees you rattling pans in the kitchen. Naps help him to keep pace with the day too. Holding it as simple as possible brings your child tremendous reassurance. They allow him to know what will happen next in his day, offering the same comfort you would get from reviewing your schedule or staring at your watch. Support your child gage a sense of time by describing sequences: "After you play, I'll pick you up, have lunch, then take a nap." "After two more nights, we'll go on holiday."

How well she remembers? More than you could imagine. While many impressions of childhood are forgotten until, we are adults, for purposes that are not entirely known, daily kids recall plenty. They can associate certain events (such as the teller gives your child a lollipop when you are going to the bank). They might start reminding themselves of the steps involved in finger painting or bedtime routine. Having a routine helps strengthen memories and builds an overall sense of security for your child. You should also motivate your child by posing him to use his recall skills: "What did we see in the zoo? "Kids prefer to usually recall things that deviate from what is planned. Therefore, instead of telling you about the lions and tigers and bears, your child might continue to talk about how he dropped his ice cream cone. In addition, Toddlers remember unusual events (such as a one-year zoo trip) more often than the routine details (say, if a zoo excursion is a regular thing). Study the day at bedtime, together. By inserting information, help your child draw on his memories: "Yes, the ice cream has dropped. Just instead, we had a pacifier! "His capacity to arrange and store memories grows dramatically as your child's language skills develop. For e.g., you may hear your child speak about a large truck he had seen two weeks earlier. Alternatively, seeing a seashell could remind him of getting a beach holiday eight months earlier. Using images also to protect memories. Hold snapshots of distant relatives available on the fridge frame, and even glance at family photos together.

How is his mind working? Toddlers are literal minds who are legendary. They lack a real understanding of the subtleties of words, meaning, and situation to see the complexities. When you say, "You are funny," your child can complain, "I'm not funny. My name is Sammy! "The child will develop more abstract thinking before age 2, as well; an illustration is the willingness to envision something that isn't there. One way that children reinforce knowing that things exist even if they are not there is by removing artifacts, and then going back to where they are placing them. Think of it as progressive peekaboo. Crackers can be found, for example, under the sofa cushions or blocks in a kitchen drawer. This lets a kid build confidence as well as an appreciation of the permanence of an object—"Is it really still there? "Exercising control is also a method of squirreling items away. Your child takes care of a tiny portion of her world in her own small way, as she chooses when. In addition, indeed, she can only wonder where those crackers are. Will he know quantity? Within his second year, your child gains knowledge of quantities in a simplistic way. A 1-year-old can understand the concept of "more," and even "big" versus "little." By age 2, your child might be able to count as accurately as two might as possible. A few bright 2-year-olds can recite their numbers from one to 10. Yet, in fact, the capacity to actually identify more than two of anything is not mastered before age 3 or older. Counting songs (such as "Ten Little Indians") is fantastic fun for children and sets the foundation for a subsequent understanding of numbers.

The sense of humor of the Children may be simplistic, but it sure does exist. Has she developed a sense of humor? Of example, satire and the stories of late-night comics go right over your child's ear. A sense of fun for a child is on the immature side. Yet there certainly is. A major game is a slapstick. Sound like sliding back, hearing your kid howl. Her weakness is confusion. For e.g., when you make your nose an elbow or claim to put a shoe on your head, infants consider it hilarious. Sometimes you can use laughter to your benefit, such as defusing a power struggle or amusing your infant when having her ready or diapered. One thumb rule: Always laugh at your wife, never at her. (Ultimately not until she will see you.)

Learning Fundamentals for Babies

A great deal of child-rearing expertise is gained at the job. Therefore, here are a few tips to burp, bathe and diaper your newborn baby.

Burping back. All babies, after being fed, will burp midway repeatedly. Burping enables unnecessary gas to exit and is swallowed through suction. The kid will keep filling faster if the air is stored in the belly; take in fewer at each meal. You can make your baby in different positions: with her looking over your shoulder, or while facing her down on your lap or sitting up. Try all of them to see which works better for your child. Using the one hand to firmly rub her back, use the other hand to protect your little one. Whereas if you make a decision to burp your child in the seated position, lean it forward, with your hand, to firmly support her head.

Sleeping

Beginning at home on the first day, placing the kid in the cradle or crib on his back while he is groggy but still conscious. This way, without any support, he can begin to drop out. Do not fret if he just is not falling asleep. You can rock him if he starts crying, but once he is calm, bring him right in the cot-before he sleeps. If he wakes up for his feedings in the middle of the night, leave the lights close to zero, and the feedings speedy and businesslike. If you start making it too pleasant, you may be encouraging more repeated feedings at night. He will have problems falling back to bed if it is too arousing.

Skin

Many newborns grow tiny white pimples on their nose and mouth, called milia, triggered by the blockage of premature oil glands. Such whiteheads vanish under their own after a few weeks. There is no need to pinch clean. Babies can also grow baby acne, triggered by hormones in their mother's body that are already circulating. The only remedy that is required is to wash the region three or four times a day with water and pat off. The pimples will disappear and leaving no visible traces in a few weeks.

Diapering

Should not use powdered pads until your baby is a couple of weeks old as it may irritate delicate skin. Alternatively, using cotton balls or a dry wipe immersed in hot water to wipe, and a warm towel or cloth to cover. Pass the powders and lotions (as lotions can irritate baby skin; the baby powder is carcinogenic and may be dangerous if babies inhale). If necessary, use cornstarch powder to keep the baby dry in warmer weather (still be careful to keep the powder distanced from her face so it will not be inhaled) and ointments only on a condition that your baby has a diaper rash. If his diaper is simply wet, no need to wash your baby at all; if it is dirty, clean extensively, always wiping from the front to the back (distant from the genitals) for hygienic reasons.

Cord Devotional Treatment

It is not necessary that you bathe your baby in a shower during the initial week or two before her umbilical cord stub dries up and falls off. A few days, a fast bubble bath is all it needs. In addition, several doctors recommend the use of newborn skin only with water. Hold the umbilical stub, where necessary, safe, open to the sun throughout the day, and disinfect that with rubbing alcohol during each change of diaper to keep it fresh and clean. When the skin across the belly button is dark or the stub starts oozing, contact the doctor.

Communication and Babies

Babies begin communication from the first day they are born. There are critical times of rapid development before formal education ever begins when the brain is finest able to obtain speech (sound development) and dialect (understanding and using words). Their communication skills are more nuanced as young children mature. They try to recognize and use language to express their feelings and thoughts and to communicate with others. Parents, family friends, and caretakers are the most critical mentors and examples of engagement for infants. However, to make the best of this crucial moment, it does not require software, videos, or any other unique resources. Your day-to-day interactions with your kids help build their brains and enable the growth of communication.

Children develop differently, but most of them follow a natural timetable for speech and language learning. Interaction milestones are skill sets that children are expected to have by some age on average. These milestones build upon each other and assist us in knowing if the stage of development is on track. Recognizing suitable communication milestones is beneficial for parents so they can promote their baby's development and seek assistance early if their toddlers do not meet them.

Expressive and Receptive Communication Skills

Babies continue learning two types of communication skills from birth: receptive skills and verbal skills.

- **Receptive communication** is the potential of a baby to accept and comprehend a message from another person. Babies exemplify this skill by shaking their heads forward into your voice and reacting, often with speech patterns, to simple directions. Early on, such vocalizations will only be sounds; however, they will start to use meaningful language as baby nears their first birthday.

- **Expressive communication** is the ability to deliver a message through noises, monologue, signs, or writing to someone else. Instances of your baby's early remarkable achievements are crying, babbling, and using body language. Below are general steps along the way for children from birth to age two to hearing, listening, speaking, language, and cognitive development. Keep in mind that development varies, and a single child may evolve better in one area than in the other. Your child may not have any of the skills mentioned before the age period is over.

First 0-3 Months

Baby will be making quiet coos and smiles at this age. Remember to communicate regularly with your baby, so they can look and learn!

4-6 Months

Although kid is not yet developing sentences, they will be responding more to your conversation. They will start making consonant sounds as well, which are the foundations for full words.

7-9 Months

Baby's range of sounds will help it rise. They would even start remembering important words, including their own titles!

10-12 Months

That is when the infant usually begins using real terms! In addition to utilizing other communication devices, they can use simple, quick terms like "mama" or "dada" to recognize their parents.

First Year

The language for the kid is increasing! They will understand many words, can use 5-10 (or more!) words alone, and respond to questions.

Second Year

The language skills of your toddler continue to advance at this age. They will start using two-word phrases by their second birthday, follow instructions, and enjoy listening to the stories

How do I know if my child has quite an error in communication?

If you notice that your child is experiencing a postponement in speech, or has any problems in comprehending communication and/or interacting with you, it is better to talk to your provider. They will help you explore other possible solutions! A speech-language pathologist is one form of healthcare provider who often struggles with communication issues. They help the kids find measures to efficiently interact through verbal and nonverbal language. If they face issues, a child may have to see a speech-language pathologist:

- Feeding or vomiting – age-appropriate meals and beverages cannot be consumed or drank safely.

- Articulating certain sonorities

- Like stuttering with fluent speech

- Difficulty utilizing words, phrases and sentences to connect at an appropriate age – require guidance use words to convey and/or turn words into phrases

- Difficulty comprehending information, such as directions or queries – needs to help you understand the words you are talking to

- Difficulty coordinating information and conduct control

- Connect to the primary provider for your child to see if a speech-language pathologist is correct for them.

1.2 Different Aspects of a Toddler's Development

Probably the most essential aspect of the schooling cycle is the first three years of life. The brain of your infant creates 700 new synaptic links every second — there is no other moment of existence when your brain is so responsive to training, or so affected by the learning experience. Harvard's Emerging Child Center considers this period of brain growth a phase of "early plasticity," which implies that the brain of your infant is easily processing the information surrounding it to build up the foundation for how it can think and respond for the remainder of their lives. The brain loses its plasticity after the first five years of life, and it gets far tougher to affect how your kids learn. For this reason, choosing a preschool for your child might be one of the most important choices you make about their academic achievement. You want to choose a curriculum that can lay the groundwork for a future of enthusiastic learning, one that will foster and direct your child as they head out on their path of school.

Infant Stimulation

There is no need to purchase or follow planned curricula aimed at improving the intellectual growth of a young child. Observe that any moment you do all of these things, you activate the consciousness of an infant:

• Love. Affection, as well as love, are needs that are very real. A small child is unaware of influencing or regulating you. She has a psychological need for your care, namely your devotion and gentle, sensitive attention. The whole compassion enables powerful self-esteem to be created and doubled brain circuitry advancement.

• Speak and sing to the kid, particularly with a nice voice, a broad range of terminology, and a lot of emotion. For example, give a remark about what you are doing while making a meal, folding laundry, or writing a grocery list. His language constructs your interactions, songs, and stories. Demonstrate emotions, shape ways of acting, and even educate problem-solving skills.

• Reply to demands from the child immediately. You do not want to try to ruin him. Not only will you pay attention to her urgent needs, but you will also teach her that she can connect with others, and her wants can be met, providing her a clear sense of confidence and emotional security and showed her that she is valuable and deserving of your love.

• Touch the baby. Keeping your kid soft, cuddling, and swaying with him, looking out for what he thinks is best. Bear in mind that showering, diapering, and milking are positions available to nurture eye contact and touch. Consider having a child in a swing or baby seat for prolonged periods.

Touch is critical to growth. For all the tactile sensations, touch is the way babies realize that they are valued first. It is comfort-source. To be held in the face of strangeness is comforting. Touch gives the brain signals asking him to expand (make connections). Without early touch fostering, it might as well be difficult for babies to survive. Babies are "massaged" when they are delivered because of the mother's bodily strength and activity. Infants need to grow that ongoing experience. Contact is a crucial resource to the brain and body alike.

Just let the child experience various surrounding environments by carrying him on family outings: to the local supermarket, the shopping center, or the park. Place him in a carriage and tour place art museums, aquariums, local restaurants, and wildlife sanctuaries. Consequently, you provide him with an exciting challenge as he experiences new sights, smells, sounds, and sensory experiences. Any excursion is enriching!

• Let the child explore differing (not too extreme) textures and temperatures. Provide a safe exploration environment, as she needs time to find things out for herself.

• Read books: reveal infants to the world of primary education early on. Although he cannot follow the story, he will love seeing pictures and your voice's sound —

In addition, it is a perfect way to communicate and strengthen the emotional connection.

• Perform music, as it stimulates and delights the senses of the child. Try to sing or play lullabies and songs, which will repeat patterns and rhythms. Attempt to walk towards the beat.

Can A Comforting Physical Touch And Assuring Eye Contact Aid In Helping Children Develop And Grow?

Children need to have a gentle touch, hold, and eye contact, just as they need food to grow and develop. Research has shown that nursing touch did help newborns put on weight and establish positive relationships with care providers, as holding and massaging an infant boosts the brain to release significant growth hormones.

• If the baby wants to be fed, hold the child. Simple indications include crying, yelling, searching for you, or staring at you.

• You can hold the infant while tending to another child's verbal needs.

• Provide the infant with other "touch" experiences, even at a very young age. Use fabrics and products, such as sheets, fluffy blankets, straw mats, etc., to position the baby on various surfaces.

• Let the baby reach various surfaces: rough, shiny, muddy, bumpy, and cold.

• Check for indicators of what type of contact the kid gloves and dislikes. Is he laughing and pretending to love the interaction, or is he fussing and turning away? Does the baby appear to hate every contact it encounters?

• Children feel things (touch) through many body parts, so rub their noses and make contact with their elbows and knees.

Six Great Strategies to Avoid Crying

Within a 24-hour cycle, infants will weep as many as 2 - 3 hours, and it is not pleasant to deal with the screeching. Use some approaches, and you can all cool down.

"To new parents, it can be overwhelming, confusing, and sometimes frightening to find out what certain screaming entails," says Rachel Alison, M.D., a family practitioner in Lexington, Kentucky co-founder of The Mommy M.D. Guide to Your Baby's First Year. "If they can't find the cause for the weeping quickly, they'll be afraid that something is medically wrong with the infant."

An inconsolable little may also render a new parent feel impotent, remarks Crystal Clancy, of Cleveland, a certified marriage and family counselor specializing in perinatal mental well-being. It can be especially distressing for women, she says, who feel confident and in charge of their pre-mom life. The positive news: You will be great at understanding and listening to the sounds of your infant, Dr. McAllister states. Put some strategies to use up to then.

1. Do the Shoosh-Bounce

Drive the munchkin in a sling, firing in her ear repeatedly. "I placed my baby in a brace and hopped her around the flat, the street, the neighborhood," says Brooklyn's Lili Zarghami. "When swinging back backward and forwards, I baked and washed."

Why It Works

"Studies show that when borne or swayed, a soothing reaction is activated in an infant's brain, allowing the baby's heart rate to slow down and the muscles to relax," says Kristie Rivers, M.D., a Fort Lauderdale podiatrist. At the same time, the shooshing sound produces a repeated diversion in which your baby can concentrate rather than scream.

Switch the Music Up

You do not need to confine only to melodies. Use the various styles and albums, just if you want. "Tom liked to hang out on Cell's 'Forget You,'" said Jennifer Louis Marquez of California. Reggae has been a preferred choice for the son of Lindsay Winston. In addition, Black Sabbath's Melanie Plea, of New York, had quite a baby with an Iron Man penchant. "He'd be giggling as long as he saw it start running," Plea says.

Why it works

Music has the ability, including action, to relax the nervous system, lowering the respiratory and heart rate of an infant. In addition, do not undervalue your own voices power-even if you are not a Taylor Swift. "Their mom's singing sound may particularly soothe infants because her tone is comfortable and the rhythm soothes," Dr. Rivers says.

Bring Lights Out

When Emily Blitzer Wildstein's children were overstimulated, she noticed that the most efficient way to soothe them was to place them in a dark space. "I'd take off dark curtains and place them with a pacifier in their bounces. The flips gave them the feeling of bouncing in our laps, so after just two minutes, they will be out like a flash," the Manhattan mom notes.

How It Tends To Work

Babies will quickly get over-stimulated by all the daily sounds and lighting. "Newborn babies are after all accustomed to the silent dim womb surroundings," Dr. Rivers notes. Obstructing all the noise will soothe them.

Make a Small Noise

Further trick parents dare say: turn white noise on. Try a fan or tumble dryer cleaner, use a machine with white noise, or download apps. The hypothesis is that such noises mimic what an infant felt in the womb when the blood of Mom flowed into the placenta, Dr. Rivers notes. White noise often hides other sounds, for example, watching siblings or packing away dishes. Only hold down on the length. Evidence suggests that devices with white noise may lead to hearing damage if they are too noisy and too near to Baby for lengthy stretches.

Keep It Up

"I'd record them fussing and crying on my phone when my sons were babies and let them listen to it. They'd been captivated by the noise of a baby crying," says Jillian Charles of Virginia.

How It Appears To Work

"Babies are so upset occasionally, they have a rough time settling down, particularly though the triggering factor, like a messy diaper, is taken good care of," Dr. Rivers says. We are practically screaming out, "stuck." A shocking diversion will jolt infants out of what gets them mad, like a video of their speech. "Babies are so involved in the environment around them, so just discovering something different will help interrupt the crying cycle," she says.

Adjust the Landscape

Jessica Brown, from Washington, swears she could notice her fussy baby as she was stressed out. "It was then I realized that it was time to turn her off to my spouse or grandparents," says the mum of three. Whereas, if she could not shift caregivers in any case, at least Brown should transfer into another area. "Perhaps it was enough to move from the bedroom to the balcony or backyard to shake her out of a weeping phase," she notes.

How It Tends To Work

"All a kid wants to improve her attitude may be a different place to reflect on," explains Dr. Rivers.

1.3 Theory of Toddler Evolution

Recent advancement in brain science has demonstrated that the environment of babies has a profound impact on brain-building and balanced growth. It is this initial phase of brain activity that predicts how one feels and learns — both as children and adults — and how well.

During the first years of a baby's life, the brain is continually building its wiring network. Brain movement produces tiny electrical associations called synapses — the number of stimuli that a child experience influences explicitly the number of synapses that develop. Repetitive and regular activation reinforces and renders the bonds lasting. We can lose some links that do not get used to it. For a young, growing brain, the early years are the "best time." This prolonged cycle of brain development and capability creation for networks happens only once in a lifetime. As careers and guardians, we have a small but rare ability to assist in promoting the brain circuitry development of our children.

Here are some interesting details discovered by researchers:

• Children have a psychological desire and an ability to know.

• The fundamental networking of brain synapses is nearly

complete within the first three years of accelerated brain growth.

• Children have a strong affinity for human appearance, expression, touch, and scent, over all others. Therefore, the best gift for the baby is you, walking, and running, handling, and talking to them.

• Fascinating stimuli may enhance excitement, focus, commitment, and the enjoyment of learning in increasing infants and babies.

• The more age-appropriate and engaging interactions, both physical and social-emotional, in which a child engages, the more circuitry will be designed to enhance learning in future.

Children go through distinctive transitional stages as they mature from babies into young adulthood. There are numerous shifts in brain growth across each of these periods. What happens and is genetically determined nearly when these developments occur. Situational conditions and interactions within the community with critical entities have a significant impact on whether growing child profits from each developmental occurrence. Stages and ages are phrases used to outline essential periods in the timeline for human development. Throughout the vital developmental realms, including the physical, psychological, language, and communication-emotional, learning and success occur at a growing stage. The aim is to help parents recognize what happens in the brain and body of their child through each time, with the expectation that they may be able to offer the required guidance, motivation, direction and strategies to allow a child to advance through each stage as quickly and effectively as possible depending on the particular collection of behaviors and desires of each individual.

Baby (Birth – 2 Years Old)

It can indeed be both difficult and fun to carry a child, especially for the first time. It is a process to grow the securities that will last a lifespan, giving the child the personal strength to build self-esteem and connect constructively to others. It is also the moment for parents to start learning who the new kid is. Each child is special, and parents must strive to recognize, appreciate, help, and foster each child's particular strengths and traits.

Toddler Development (18 Months-3 Years)

A new stage of testing starts when a kid takes its first steps. Children during this stage are free to roam around their environment. This is an opportunity to deliberately discover their settings. The development of language is growing significantly, leading to the teaching of the names of points of interest, the capacity to ask for things. As they find their independence, yes, they grow the ability to say, "No! "The creation of what psychologist's term emotional control is a major problem during this developmental period. At this time, "Meltdowns" are regular, but parents may use the relationship formed through childhood to help them learn to amplify their emotional communication and begin to understand the complicated concept of delay of gratification. Although they tend to be able to answer "Yes," spontaneously, children do require guidance, understanding how to embrace "Yes" from others. This is also a phase of rapid intellectual and social development, readying these children to start kindergarten, which includes collaborative interaction with peers while being able to compete emotionally and cognitively at the same time. The parent of a child is in a situation to be a coach that provides the right mix of encouragement, support, and guidance. Parents will always function as the principal tutor for the mastering of fundamental skills and promote constructive exploration and testing with novel ideas and abilities.

How Toddlers Play

Do children of various development planes behave differently? Yes. In addition, understanding these stages would be helpful for you so that you can encourage your child to learn through his play. Here is how it breaks down:

• 12-18 months old: A young toddler explores with her hands through her senses and manipulates items. She tests how one behavior causes another (for starters, throwing out all the toys in a bucket just to see if they fall). Your house is her sandbox, as she uses her new walking, running, and roaming skill. Her play is loose and unstructured but she will look for guidance to an adult. She wants support so she only keeps fine-tuning her eye-hand synchronization, excellent motor abilities, and finger function.

• 18-24 months old: As big and tiny muscle abilities grow, a kid puts things where he needs them to go and uses trial and error to solve challenges (example: solving a basic wooden jigsaw puzzle. He is going to run and go up there. He pretends more and he performs activities that he sees grown-ups do. He works alone, or with a parent. However, he is still not going to play with other men.

• Age two years. A two-year-old loves playing. She creates a story or plays

Toy or toy condition (such as driving racing cars or having a baby doll on a stroll). Adults help by taking on a role or giving the event's play-by-play. Her developed little muscle skills have helped her to handle objects, draw, and paint. She should start building things up. A two-year-old works with another infant and takes care of what the infant does. Two-year-olds still do not play together.

• Age three years. A three-year-old is great at getting limited body abilities. That, and his improved reasoning abilities, let him play some sophisticated games. He-order or series objects, string beads, or work out a more complex puzzle. He is already more organized, suggesting he will appreciate more playground games. And three-year-olds like playing together (in the end you can take a break from being the only playmate for your child!).

• Aged four years. A four-year-old works regularly with other children — and much of that is creative play. For make-believe situations, every kid has a role to play. He should enjoy the park and early sporting activities as he has excellent body strength and strong balance. A four-year-old may have great little coordination abilities, so they can start writing

letters and cutting with scissors. Others are also focusing on those credentials.

Importance of Play

A fascinating research looked at the impact of children (aged 18-30 months) with autism and caregivers who utilized "play-based" coping methods to interact with them. Half of the children sought expert treatment. The other group had therapy with professionals and their parents, who learned how to use specific teaching strategies at home. Two years after the professional-only party saw a seven-point rise in IQ scores. The community of children who have both specialists and qualified parents working for them has seen a rise in IQ points of 17.6 percent. (Dawson G) While this study specifically tackled autism children and parents who were taught how to play with their children, consider the wider implications. You might think it is just game time to sit down with your kid to have a tea party or construct a Lego tower. Yet practicing social awareness, listening abilities, eye-hand coordination, relational connections, counting, and organizing is an important moment for an infant. You can help guide your child's play to make him consider these things.

Preschooler Growth

The preschoolers emerge from childhood into a modern era of adventure and structured schooling. Most have begun or will begin pre-school or pre-kindergarten and will end this development duration before starting formal school in either nursery school or first grade. Since pre-school has been more precise and mostly incorporates what was once first grade, kids typically begin kindergarten about six years of age. Kindergartners are open to numbers, letters, reading starts, and simple math. It is always a crucial moment for music listening. We are enhancing the gross motor and motor skill capabilities, which keeps them involved in drawing, crafts, and all sorts of ride-on toys (cars, scooters, motorcycles, etc.). Children are learning new athletic abilities, sometimes contributing to interest in competitive sports even by the end of this phase of growth. During this period, the most critical way of teaching is play. Make sure play of all sorts is alluring and encourages language acquisition, social interaction, and creative thinking. An early passion for science promotes interest in pursuing their environment. They always like to create stuff around the house from objects as well as construction sets like Legos, Kenexa, blocks, and others.

1.4 Sensory Activities for Your Toddler's Brain Development

Our brains are composed of trillions of brain cells, called neurons, and connections, called synapses, among them. The first three years are the time a baby's brain is growing at a fast rate. While a child is born with approximately 50 trillion synapses, the brain of a three-year-old has grown to 1000 trillion.

Senses contribute to the multiple ways we experience the universe. Our brains use many senses to help us maneuver within our surroundings. Taste, smell, sight, touch, and sound are the five most commonly recognized senses. Children use their five senses from conception to early adolescence to investigate and attempt to make sense of the environment around them. It's an essential part of their early childhood development. It is crucial for brain development to provide opportunities for children to actively use their senses as they explore their world through 'sensory play.' Learning through sensory exploration naturally comes to infants and small children. Now that makes sense when you consider that the skill sets they will continue to depend on to build comprehension of objects, spaces, individuals, and encounters are yet to be fully mature. Our senses, as adults, send us crucial knowledge that we use to guide decision-making countless times a day. It is likely that we take this ability for granted and barely notice it, but it is for that reason that it is so important to help children learn about their senses. In essence, infants participate in a sensory activity whenever they move, jump, touch, taste, hear, see, and smell. However, with the activities that are shared below, you may give them a mega-dose of sensory uplift.

Why Should Toddlers Attempt Sensory Activities

You might wonder why it is essential, and that is a reasonable question. The possible explanation you see sensory activities while scrolling through Facebook is because it dramatically boosts brain function and development by stimulating the senses that occur during those activities. That is even more effective when children, like infants, engage in them at an early age.

As intriguing as it may sound, sensory activities can help them to be better readers in the toddler years and to attend well when they are down the road in school years.

From conception to early adolescence, infants use their senses to discover their environment and seek to make sense. They do so by holding, smelling, tasting, seeing, running, and listening. Children or even grown-ups tend to learn better when engaging with most of their senses and preserve the most data. Most of our favorite moments are correlated with some or all of our senses: for example, the smell of a campfire summer night or a melody you memorized with a school friend to the lyrics. Now, when those commonly associated smells and sounds stimulate your nostrils and eardrums, respectively, your brain forces and recall a memory flashback to those special times. Giving opportunities for

children to effectively use their sensory perception as they start exploring their world through 'sensory play' is essential for brain development – it helps build nerve connections in brain pathways. This adds to the capacity of a child to perform increasingly challenging learning activities, which encourages academic growth, language acquisition, gross motor skills, social engagement, which problem-solving abilities.

However, Sensory Activities Are More Essential for Some Toddlers

Besides being fantastic for overall development sensory activities for toddlers, some kids might need them. Some children search for senses more than the average boy searches, or fear sensations. That is not a negative thing, although it may conflict with their capacity to perform tasks that need to be accomplished by children. For example, in children, sensory problems can sound like difficulties stopping one task and beginning another (conversion). Alternatively, if they step barefoot inside the field, go down a drop, or feel a squishy substance, they can freak out. On the other hand, your child could also be ferocious, climb the bedding, and make the bunny energizer look like a slow tortoise in motion.

Sensory Playing benefits

There is always a lot more happening with sensory play than it meets the eye. As well as being enjoyable and engaging for infants and small children, interactive experiences allow them to learn and study. In addition, these activities aid children in using the 'scientific method' of observing, hypothesizing, experimenting, and drawing conclusions.

Sensory activities also allow kids to optimize their threshold values for different sensory information, helping their brain build better connections to sensory information, and learning, which is helpful and which can be filtered out. For example, when there is too much happening in their environment with conflicting noises or sights, a child may find it hard to play with other children. Through sensory play, the child can take lessons to block out the unnecessary noise and concentrate on the play that is taking place with their peer. Another instance is a toddler who is notably fussy eating foods such as spaghetti with a wet texture. In an atmosphere of no anticipation, the usage of tactile play will enable the child to reach, feel, and interact with the material. As the child develops confidence and understanding of this texture, it helps build positive brain pathways to say, engaging in this food is safe.

Sensory Function Is Not All About Touch

Some people automatically imagine sand and water tables or children playing with mud and playdough when they think about tactile play, but it is not just about touch; it is about the other senses too. For example, the dramatic scent of lemon juice involved in a science project, the color schemes of water during a color blending experiment, or the scratch and sniff painting texture. Smells are all portion of catering to your child's senses. Tactile learning is a means for children to explore, learn, categorize, and make sense of the environment, and it is important to provide them chances for a sensory activity.

Sensory Language Abilities

Playing with various kinds of textures, flavors, and objects help your child develop new ways to talk about the world. The forest is simply more than a vine, a sapling with smooth bark, or a pine tree with a rugged bark and a strong pine smell. The liquid is not only warm, but it may also be rugged (waves), bubble-slippery, or icy and transparent until frozen. Flavors, too, could even build the base of language for your kid. She does not want potato chips for dinner anymore, so she needs something tangy or spicy or nice, so definitely not sour or bland.

Sensory Practice Is Calm

You might have found that your child seems calmer after a bath or that your child is more settled after an especially rough session of running around the house, knocking in furniture, falling into his bed, or pillows. Such a form of tactile activity is soothing for infants, as it allows them to control their inner distress, be it anxiety, restlessness, or some other sort of frustration.

Regulating Actions and Feelings

Other forms of tactile play may be soothing and help a child control. Heavy job, sensory feedback affecting the sensory system of proprioception, may be particularly successful in controlling behavior. Focusing on a relaxing experience may help relieve a child's anxiety, mainly if it is an experience devoted to relaxation like one that includes the fragrance of lavender.

It Improves Exceptional Motor Abilities.

The kind of action happening in sensory play such as squishing, pinching, sorting, placing, and scooping is designed to enhance motor coordination skills and increase coordination.

The Curiosity In Learning Flares

Adding sensory elements to instruction can improve a child's attention and can stimulate a learning interest. Children who learn through play enjoy themselves more and want to do more of it. There are several opportunities to integrate tactile activity into instruction.

Chapter 2: Fundamentals of Montessori Method of Learning

Montessori is a Children's Schooling methodology. It is a place for children to look at and recognize. This is a perception of the growth and learning of children, which has been transformed into a comprehensive form of education focused on rigorous empirical research. This is focused on self-directed thinking, hands-on training, and engaging in a partnership. Kids make imaginative decisions in their learning at the Montessori classes, whilst the curriculum and the professionally qualified instructor provide age-appropriate tasks to direct the method. Children work in teams to uncover and explore world knowledge individually, and to evolve to their full potential. The Montessori academic structure is complex in that it has been successfully undergoing development process for over a hundred years, and was used effectively in various regions around the world with children of all levels and ages, including diverse and greater pace. Perhaps the most important explanation for its popularity is that it is a holistic instructional system arising from the convergence of growth, learning, instruction, and teaching science.

2.1 The History of Montessori

Maria Montessori currently receives widespread recognition as one of the best educators in the country. Her life story is incredible — one where a committed woman used her scientific background, her expertise, and observations to establish an educational method that defied conventional educational trends. The traditions that she defied were not only intellectual ones: she needed to tackle the barriers that hindered women's ability to pursue different professions. Montessori was born in a small city Chiaravalle, overlooking the Adriatic Sea, in the province of Ancona in Italy, on August 31, 1870; she was the only born of a highly respected family's well-educated daughter Alessandro Montessori, a businessperson in the country's tobacco monopoly; and mother, Renilde Stoppani. Maria Montessori was born under the House of Savoy, hardly ten years after the unification of Italy. During the "Risorgimento," headed by a moderate political leader, Camillo Cavour, and a fiery nationalist, Giuseppe Garibaldi, in 1871, the minor parties and city-states on the Italian peninsula eventually unified as one nation. The Carbonari, the red-shirted volunteer army of Giuseppe Garibaldi, had overthrown the former bourbon monarchy of the "Two Sicilies" and the forces of Piedmont-Sardinia had taken Victor Emmanuel as constitutional monarch to the Italian throne.

In the year 1896, Montessori became the first woman to qualify from the Medical Department of the University of Rome and joined the staff of the Psychological Clinic of the university. She accompanied the girls confined to the chronically insane asylums in Rome as part of her duties there. She was aware that such intellectually driven children could benefit from special education and flew to London and Paris to research the work of Jean Itard and Edouard Seguin, two early leaders in this eld. Upon her return, Montessori was asked by the Italian Minister of Education to give the Rome teachers a lecturing course. The course grew into the State Orthophrenic Academy, and in 1898, Montessori was named its director.

For two years, she interacted with the kids there, basing her methods of education on the experiences she had learned from Itard and Seguin. All-day, 8:00 A.M. She taught at the school until 7:00 P.M. and then worked far into the night to plan new materials, make notes and discoveries, and respond to her work. She found these two years to be her "real degree" in college. To her astonishment, she realized these kids being willing to know certain items that appeared unlikely. The first class of Dr. Maria Montessori started in 1907 and composed of around 50 to 60 children, ages 3 to 6, who grew up in the slums of Rome, Italy. Maria characterized the periods between three and six years as an especially sensitive time in which young children are proactively reaching to knowledge acquisition from and about their surroundings.

Dr. Montessori established a "prepared environment" of child-sized furnishings to adapt the surroundings to the original size and behavior of the child, to enrich their experience. This did help the kids feel comfortable and relaxed, and the atmosphere dramatically increased their interest in learning. She also established hands-on teaching programs that had been developed logically. The students developed an extraordinarily high degree of cognitive and social capability at young ages through their observations and interactions in this structured environment. The news of Dr. Montessori's unprecedented success in his work at this 'Casa Dei Bambini' (Children's House) quickly spread worldwide, and people came from far away lands and wide to observe for themselves the exclusive educational advances of these children. The famous Glass Classroom of Dr. Maria Montessori at the Panama-Pacific World Fair in San Francisco, 1915. In the back of the room is Dr. Montessori wearing a feathered hat.

About Casa Dei Bambini

The Casa Dei Bambini a motivating force in the career of Montessori came in 1907 when Edoardo Talamo requested her to create a school in Rome's slum area. Now, Talamo was managing director of the Institute de Romano di Beni Stabili (the Better Building Association), a charitable association founded to enhance poor people's housing conditions. The organization acquired and remodeled takedown, overcrowded, and unhygienic tenements in the city. It has been engaged in the housing recovery in the quarter of San Lorenzo, a neighborhood of Rome affected by poverty. The invitation Talamo made to Montessori was an effort to reconcile a very practical issue. As parents who stayed in redeveloped housing went to college, their children were left isolated and unmonitored at kindergarten. With these babies, the association agreed to create the school as some kind of daycare center. Nevertheless, Montessori has already had the ability to build a school that will act as a classroom for exploring her theories. John Dewey, too, was studying his theoretical theories at the University of Chicago Laboratory School is much more suitable conditions. In both educators' situations, such educational studies will create their identities as leading educators. On January 6, 1907, Montessori initiated her first-ever school, the Casa Dei Bambini, or Children's House, in a large property on Via Dei Marsi, in the poverty-ridden district of San Lorenzo, Rome. Her first pupils were fifty girls, between the ages of three and seven, whose parents resided in the house.

The Children's House was built educationally to be a classroom-home, an academic entity in close vicinity to the families of children. In reality, it was in the apartment where the kids lived. Montessori said, "We brought the school inside the building. The education would lead to the socialization of the father and the workplace, which would result in effect bind the workplace with the wider community. The real physical relation of the children's home to education has a socio-economic aspect connected to the Montessori concept of the 'modern woman' of the 20th century. However, Montessori proposed that in the future, not only working-class women should be hired outside the house, but also more people of all social backgrounds should enter the workplace. The guiding force in putting about this shift in women's employment was mechanization and technical progress. Schools, as academic institutions, required to acknowledge this technologically produced change to provide for working mother children. Schools such as the Casa Dei Bambini would allow mothers to leave their children safely and "continue their own work with an emotion of great relief and freedom." following the difference in work arrangements and destinations, Montessori recommended that mothers would still have the greatest responsibility for the physical plus psychological care of their own children. The Casa Dei Bambini will help them discharge these parental obligations when seeking jobs and leisure outside the home.

In 1913, the highly regarded Alexander Graham Bell invited Dr. Montessori to the United States. Thomas Edison, Helen Keller, and others were among Montessori's supporters excited about the new Method of education. That year Alexander Graham Bell and his father established the Montessori Educational Association, with Alexander Graham Bell as its Leader. Dr. Montessori was invited to take part in the World's Fair Panama-Pacific International Exhibition, which was held in San Francisco during her second visit to the U.S. in 1915, gaining world attention with her classroom exhibit "glass house." She established a lecture hall at the Panama-Pacific Exhibition in San Francisco, where viewers watched twenty-one kids, all fresh to this Montessori Method, four months behind the same glass wall in what is now known as the Glass Classroom. The only two gold medals granted for education ended up going to this class, and the schooling of young children was forever altered.

That being said, after new fervent support for the Montessori educational Method, educational specialists in the U.S. chose to progress a different way in the American public schools. Thus, the Montessori Method at that time did not extend in the U.S.A. and rather developed more than that in Europe and other parts of the world. That momentous intention to accept a different model for education in America today has led to what is now the frequently derided educational atmosphere and conditions prevailing today in schools in the United States. Many advocates for education now acknowledge the weak points of the adopted conventional American system. Many in schooling and government have authorized repeated appeals for reform of culture and revamp of the country's education system.

A female teacher called Nancy McCormick Rambusch began searching for solutions to the conventional American education in 1953. Her quest led her to Paris to speak with Mario Montessori, the child of Dr. Maria Montessori, who had been her successor and pioneer of the Montessori Community, at the Tenth International Montessori Conference. Mario urged Rambusch to take up the Montessori education coursework and bring this same Montessori Method to the United States. Rambusch embraced this idea, and in a few years, she was in her New York City apartment trying to conduct Montessori classes with her children and others. In September 1958, she opened the Whit by School in Greenwich, Connecticut, in cooperation with a cohort of influential Catholic families.

By 1960, an American rebirth of Montessori education, with Nancy McCormick Rambusch as one of its early leaders, began to take shape. What accompanied was the advancement of the American Montessori motion, with various supporters, representatives, and organizations from Montessori, high-quality teacher structural model across the state. In the year 1976, a group of Montessori teachers met by establishing the Louisiana Montessori Association (L.M.A.) to unite their efforts to support Montessori education in Louisiana. That same year, when the Louisiana legislative body permitted the L.M.A. to certify non - government Montessori teachers and schools in Louisiana, Louisiana increased awareness of US Montessori education.

The work of Dr. Maria Montessori is enduring. In 1907 in Rome, the initial Casa Dei Bambini launched. Today,

Montessori teaching proceeds in hundreds of educational institutions around the U.S. and across the globe. For Montessori schools in at least 110 cities, this is worldwide in nature. Montessori schools can be used in agricultural, urban, and city best; in middle-class towns, affluent neighborhoods, and even remote villages. Montessori was a good catholic, and she remained steeped in religion in all of her teachings. She saw the kid as being spiritual. For training for adulthood, Dr. Maria Montessori worked for the best possible creation of the human capacity. She saw teaching as a conceptual model where the child's core character has to deeply participate. To educate the entire child, she concluded that to develop emotionally, physically, intellectually, and spiritually the child must be given freedom. Montessori discovered that the only vital impulse to learn is the children's self-motivation, and without it, the child effectively ceases to learn. The teacher provides the climate, directs the actions, acts as the guidance, and provides stimulation for the child. Then the instructor remains back and watches while the infant starts to show itself by "practice," which is the driving factor behind the kid's search for information.

More about the Sensitive Stages

Montessori witnessed Sensitive stages in the life of the infant relating to a desire for harmony in the world, the usage of the hands and mouth, the progress of the movement, an obsession for a minute and informative items, and a phase of deep social involvement.

Order is the first Sensitive Time to turn up. This occurs early, also in the first months, in the first year of existence, and lasts into the second year. It is important to note that Montessori saw a strong difference between the enjoyment of order and discipline of the infant and the milder joy and happiness of the experienced individual in getting this in place. The love of the child's order is based upon an essential need for an accurate and defined atmosphere. The child may categorize his experiences only in such a context, thus creating an inner mental structure to grasp and interact in his universe. It is not things in the position that he recognizes through his unique attention to order, however the interaction between things. He has an inner meaning, not a way of discriminating between objects, but interprets an entire world of interconnected elements. It is only in such a setting, recognized as a whole that the child may organize himself and behave purposefully; because without it, he will have a little foundation on which to construct his understanding of the relationship. The boy demonstrates to us his need for order in three ways: he displays an intense pleasure in having objects in their normal position; he sometimes gets confused when they are not; even when he can do it himself, he may focus on placing items back in their area.

A second receptive phase emerges as an urge to discover the world with tongue, even paws. The infant learns the characteristics of the items in his atmosphere through taste and contact and tries to act upon them. Equally critically, the neural mechanisms for language are formed via this sensory-motor operation. Therefore, Montessori believed that the tongue that man uses to talk and the hands that he uses for practice is more closely connected to his intellect than any other body component. She named them the "instruments" for the intellect of man. In this Sensitive Time, the infant will be introduced to the language, or it will not grow. Itard's portrayal of Aveyron's "wild child" is probably the most profound depiction of such an occurrence. Abandoned as a baby in the mountains of France, the boy was discovered in early manhood, perhaps only in his twenties. Coated with scars from his survival in the wilderness, his moves and behavior were an animal's. Itard has been able to help this kid develop his human life potential in nearly every way.

Nonetheless, the boy did not acquire language, although it

was identified that the boy was not deaf and that there was no other defect that could obstruct lingual development. Throughout our society, the infant is generally accompanied by the noises he wants to build meaning. During this Delicate Time, through use of his hands is always another issue, even though it is equally essential to his growth. To build his neurological frameworks for vision and learning, he must have stimuli to study even as he requires to be introduced to the environment of human speech to improve his neurological structures for expression. Adult objects typically engulf the child during this time. "The 'don't reach' sign! 'It is the only solution to the critical childhood development issue. If the child approaches these prohibited things, he is disciplined or scolded. "It is, therefore, necessary to note that the infant's acts are not the product of an arbitrary decision but are driven by his inner behavioral needs. "Therefore, the actions of the infant are not down to chance. He constructs the required actions for coordinated activities driven by his ego, which orders from inside." Hence, it is crucially important that the individual is led by patience and knowledge while putting some appropriate limits on the ability of the child to touch and taste throughout this time. The most easily recognized individual is undoubtedly the Prone Time for Moving. This time Montessori considered the infant as a second birth, for it hailed his transformation from a powerless person to an active person. Older people do not remember one reality found by Montessori during this time: kids want to go for lengthy walks at this period. Montessori discovered that children as small as one and a half years old would travel many miles without exhaustion.

A fourth Critical Time includes an increased curiosity in items that are so small and complex; they can totally avoid our attention. Tiny creatures barely recognizable to the naked eye will consume the child. It is as though she is putting apart a unique time to discover and enjoy her secrets, which a distracted person might later forget. A fifth Sensitive Time is exposed by involvement in living social facets. The kid is actively interested in recognizing other people's human rights and building a relationship for them. He seeks to practice etiquette and to support himself and others. Such mutual interaction is initially displayed as an expression of curiosity, which then grows into a preference for more direct communication with others. Montessori as one of her most significant achievements and their further research to be an important challenge for educators regarded her development of the Sensitive Periods. The rules regulating the setting up of developmental development had been entirely unexplained until these discoveries of real child-nature. Studying the Critical Periods as guiding man's creation could become one of the sciences with the greatest practical value to humanity.

The Sensitive Periods outline the scope that the infant observes when thinking about his surroundings. The Absorbent Mind phenomena describe the unique nature and mechanism through which he fulfills the awareness. As the mind of the infant is not yet established, he will learn from the individual in a different manner. The adult individual has an awareness of his world to draw on, but the kid has to continue with zero. It is the Consuming Mind, which fulfills this apparently insurmountable mission. It allows for an involuntary uptake of the environment through a special pre-conscious mental state. Through such a process, the infant explicitly integrates information into his mental existence. "Perceptions do not only invade his consciousness, but they also shape it, they are personified in him." This trains the subconscious for an unnoticed task. It is "succeeded by a rational cycle that gradually awakens and removes what it canoer from the unconscious." That way, the infant develops his mind until, bit by bit, he has developed awareness, the capacity to learn, and the ability to think.

The implicit planning needed for the subsequent development and operation is developed by the age of three. Now the infant embarks on a new journey, improving its mental functions. "The roles are produced before three; they grow after three." The Montessori theory also suggests that the infant possesses a "spiritual fetus" or cycle of psychological growth just before conception. Unless this embryo is to grow according to its design, the two aspects of an integrated interaction with the world and the independence for the infant must remain. The child's aim is to grow better, and he is naturally guided against this objective with an unprecedented strength in development. The values or universal rules that control the spiritual growth of the infant manifest themselves only through its evolutionary cycle. Through providing the Casa Dei Bambini's children an accessible atmosphere in which to act, Montessori was willing to experience certain universal laws at a function in the children and allow the start of their association with them.

Montessori Wins Educational Reputation

By 1910, Dr. Montessori had gained prominence in her homeland Italy as a significant creative instructor, where she ruled over a model school and a directresses training college. Her increasing popularity gained attention in academic settings in other E.U. countries as well as in North America, particularly in the U.S. At this stage, she addressed the question of whether her approach can be circulated and legitimized. Educational innovators also recruit followers who are energetic and well intentioned but who are untrained or poorly disciplined. They also misinterpret things because they are away from both the visionary and the heart of creativity. Montessori also needed to make several crucial choices about whether to preserve and transmit her revolutionary process. She was desperate to hold firm control in her own grip. She should monitor Montessori educators' preparation to prevent any divergence from her system as she formulated it. She will monitor the development and delivery of resources and regimes from Montessori. Her judgment will have serious repercussions for the Montessori process. Montessori utilized two proven ways of dispersing her approach to meet a broader audience: communication skills and publishing. Montessori was an expert speaker as a university educator, and she made use of speaking in public to her benefit. Her 1913 American tour is an indication of her usage of the public stage to introduce her approach to a larger audience. Again, Montessori was often qualified as a university lecturer at using journals to disseminate her theories to both trained educators and the community. She wrote in The Form of

Experimental Pedagogy Related to Infant Learning in Children's Houses in 1910 about her research at the Casa Dei Bambini. Scientific Pedagogy was written in eleven countries, renamed The Montessori Approach (1912). Dr. Montessori's Own Manual (1914) was accompanied by the Montessori Approach, which she published as a type of formal introduction to the system that would differentiate it from those who were speaking on Montessori schooling. Her work of two-volumes, the enhanced Montessori Method, emerged in 1918 and 1919. Nevertheless, papers are subject to thorough analysis in the world of academic theory and practice, particularly in higher education. Nevertheless, Montessori became mainly concerned with spreading her approach as she had thought of it rather than participating in the wider dialogue and discussion on schooling

It is important to provide longevity over time in terms of reinforcing an invention, such that it has an existence that stretches past that of its original author. Montessori switched on instructor preparedness to maintain her approach to ensure it was implemented without exaggeration. She set up a vocational school to educate directress Montessori. A Trainee who traveled all the way ecstatically from America to

Italy described Montessori as "an influential and magical personality who has the ability to make her words appear to be winged carriers of light and the mighty hold of enthusiasm is phenomenal to the beholder." Montessori trainees were mostly young women with an interest in music and art but attracted to education. Elementary instruction became heavily feminized throughout the early twentieth century, and Montessori education's tendency to draw women to its membership was to be anticipated, as the Montessori schools were early childhood institutions, usually taught by females. The bond between Montessori and her trainees has been that of the mother-leader. The pupils had become followers of her. She wanted those she trained as directresses, requiring obedience and devotion, to maintain the system in its original nature, as she had planned it.

A hallmark of Montessori's teacher training methodology was that the technique could be studied and applied without deviating from the initial template. Although this ensured conceptual accuracy, it generated several significant barriers to its propagation. First, it was said that there would be a restricted number of directresses as Montessori regulated their teaching with such rigor. Moreover, concerns concerning the need to reformulate the process to improve its validity in various historical and ethnic settings have emerged.

The Method as Academic Theory and Practice

As you might have read above, Montessori's educational Method was laid on her conceptualization of science, her children's observations, and her thorough research in anthropology, psychology, and teaching methods. Through study and practice, she, therefore, came up with a number of "discoveries" or observations on the development, growth, and education of children. To explore her system, we continue with Montessori's perception of the child's existence as a learner.

While Montessori's definition of infant development was mystical, indeed, even supernatural, treating her approach as "rational pedagogy." Every child at birth, she claimed, acquires telekinetic abilities, and internal self-teacher that boosts learning. Innately children experience the inherent capacity of consuming and integrating multiple aspects of a diverse society without formal guidance. Having reached into the transcendent to describe her concept of the nature of children, Montessori wanted to move away from abstract generalizations of philosophy to the use of the scientific theory to discover the patterns of development of children. In doing so, she was able to structure a learning environment and a set of formative assessment that fully accentuated human development patterns. The instructional Method, for Montessori, accepted two main and essential aspects: the particular child and the climate. The key component is the mental and physiological nature of the individual student, which gives him or her the power to act. The biological child has a body as an actual physical entity, a physiological framework that develops, but each kid also has a spiritual side, a psychic form that expresses itself. The atmosphere offers the required setting in which the individual being evolved, the supplementary dimension. While the world the infant inhabits will alter growth, the basic mental and physical structure of an individual being can never be developed. Education of the child needs an environment in which they can create the powers nature gives. Schooling then is a cooperative effort with the nature of the child and developmental stages. Kids respond to events and circumstances found in the world by their contact and engagement with the world. The bodily and spiritual forces of children push them to free play in their study of the world. All these experiences and the knowledge they carry with them are integrated into the creation of the child's self, understanding, and mental network. This is important that children behave openly in their environment. Their free activity reveals to the educator the signs of child development, resulting in the inventions that enable a method of instruction to be designed. Unlike standard educators who assumed that kids require shaping their interests for them, Montessori asserted that children naturally had a strong propensity and mental concentration capacity. However, the secret to practicing this personality-activity originated from internal influences rather than from exterior to the infant. If they were genuinely engaged in their sport, kids would center their time and resources on that. They would stick with it and keep working on it until they had perfected it.

2.2 Comparison between Montessori and Traditional Learning

A Montessori program is focused mostly on well-researched children's learning concepts. It incorporates a curriculum built on hands-on tools and experiences that help a child develop a positive self-image, high standards of academic and non-academic skills, and trust in the difficulties. Conventional schooling is profoundly rooted in the notion of structured learning as a mass development. The common idea specifies that everyone will know the same lessons simultaneously; nevertheless, one of Montessori education's main benefits is flexibility and customization.

Montessori-educated children, motivated to investigate and analyze from an early age, are problem-solvers and critical thinkers who handle their time and collaborate well with others. They openly share thoughts and speak about jobs. This is typically anticipated that children in a typical daycare, nursery, or preschool setting would advance in a group-driven program in a teacher-centered atmosphere with little too little ability to direct their education according to their talents, preferences, to skills. Guided by professionally qualified and professional instructors, learners in Montessori schools can dig deeper into themes and issues of common interest while seeking to follow a Montessori curriculum's rigorous academic expectations.

Montessori Is Kids Centered Learning

The greatest difference of the Montessori philosophy is its focus on becoming child-centered. So what does this signify? All children grow in different velocities, and they have unique attributes and different interests. While every kid in the class has to follow one plan set out by the instructor in traditional education, a Montessori education uses the method of observation to follow the preferences of the individual child.

The Curriculum Can Be Adapted

Every single child is different. The adaptable curriculum of Montessori schools reflects that fact by letting each child go at their own pace. Each age bracket (0-3 years, 3-6, 6-9 years, etc.) has distinct educational objectives, which are guided by each student. Learners can choose what lecture they want to learn, and over time, teachers observe students to assess their progress. The traditional curriculum, by contrast, involves a distinct path that all students should follow.

The Montessori Classroom Organized Décor Calms

Space is split into five focus areas of the Montessori Pre-school classroom: Practical Life, English, Math, Sensorial Learning, and History & Sciences. This same classroom is structured and uncluttered in order to avoid distortion and to underline that this is a learning area. Whereas traditional classrooms use vivid colors, banners, and decorations to try as well as energize children, classrooms at Montessori aim to encourage the minds of children with performance lessons.

Disruptions Are Relatively Low

Because teachers at Montessori regard the model, they honor the absorption of a child. If a student is deeply involved in their lesson, the teachers will allow them to complete what they are working on. Unlike conventional classrooms whereby children are guided to any task irrespective of their degree of interest, Montessori prevents as far as necessary interrupting the routine of the children.

Lectures are hands-on

Students actively participate in their education, instead of sitting ineffectively during the lectures. They have the duty to address the subjects that they are involved in, and they are highly engaged in the lessons by design. The lectures also consist of interactive objects for Montessori nursery classes — children will be practically "hands-on" for math and communication abilities.

Teachers Montessori Accompany the Children

Instead of training an infant for the school, the teachers plan the child's school. Montessori teachers reveal the inherent ability of any child by watching children and taking care of their desires and stages of comprehension. They keep records of progress, preparation, and topic interests so that when

planning the curriculum for the day, they can rely on the information later on.

Montessori Supports Afflicted or Children on the Autistic Continuum

Kids with ADHD or adolescents on an autism disorder excel in fixed plan conditions. Luckily, although the training at Montessori is adaptable, the everyday schedule is relatively constant. As described before, the Montessori classroom is far more structured than the traditional American pre-school classroom and has few disruptions. The Montessori theory of modeling actions often helps children on the continuum or with ADHD. Since empathy and cognitive awareness are part of the de facto program, children with autism should be best suited for social interaction.

Outdoor Space Is Accessible For Reading As Well

Outdoor time is called "recess" in traditional schools because it is a change from lessons. However, learning can be fun in itself, in the Montessori setting. Montessori children should see it as an expansion of the curriculum rather than treating outside play as a diversion from schooling. Gardening, natural reading fields, and interactive math resources are only a handful of children's enriching and engaging outdoor

experiences to enjoy.

Montessori Facilitates Children to Learn To Love

The children learn how to take tests in the traditional classroom. However, they cultivate a lifelong enjoyment of learning in kids in the Montessori classroom, so that they can appreciate and respect their education, particularly in later life. The lessons in themselves are not compulsory. Instead, students are able to tackle different topics they like to know the most. Teachers offer options to the learners so that they have personal control when being guided.

Respect & Mindfulness

Telling etiquette and principles to children requires so much more than simply teaching them to say "please" and "thank you." Teachers at Montessori recognize that children are still studying them, and they are modeling positive conduct to encourage them in their pupils. Montessori principle adults will also behave because they wish the children to act —respectful and conscious of the emotions of others. Montessori instructors often explore the emotions of children and improve their social maturity, in addition to teaching positive behavior. They ask factors that allow kids to learn to have compassion and empathy. To put it plainly, "thank you" and

"sorry" are not sufficient for a Montessori kid. They have to recognize the meaning behind these terms, too.

Montessori Schools thrive A Love For lessons

In addition, if you take a kid to school each day, you cannot push them to know. If you want your kid to get the most out of their time at the school, you need to make them feel excited about learning. This is what all teachers at Montessori do. Teachers at Montessori enjoy what they do, so they will try to pass the passion on to their pupils. When a pupil heads to a Montessori program, they are not just going to continue to study at classes; they are going to be searching for information on their own time.

Students Are Told How to Correct Themselves

Public schools waste a great deal of energy, controlling students' behavior. Your instructors and other school administrators are actively warning pupils. They are given a more critical ability when a kid goes to a Montessori high. Instead of punishing an infant, the resources it requires to correct itself are provided to a kid. A kid should be able to modify his / her actions in time. Students must have to accept and benefit from their errors.

Students and Parents Are Members of the Community with Close Partnerships

Montessori classrooms are tiny, so this means they are near to the individuals attending the classes. When a kid joins a Montessori curriculum, they must learn with the same people for at least three years and interact with the same educators. Near relations should grow throughout this period.

One of the aspects a Montessori school aims to do is to imitate a family's arrangement. When a kid goes to a Montessori school, no matter where they are, they will feel like they are being supported. There is a lot of kids who dread going to school. Kids that go to Montessori colleges, however, are typically enthusiastic about going to college. They absolutely cannot wait to get to see their educators and friends. The results of the classroom Montessori are evident. If you want to make the best possible start in life for your child, consider enrolling them in a Montessori education program. Some of the country's sharpest students began their education using a Montessori school. Start the same way with your kids.

How Differs Montessori from a Daycare Centre

Checking at various childcare choices for your kid, you may find that there are several main distinctions in a Montessori nursery that set it apart from your typical daycare. Each classroom in a preschool in Montessori is unique, even though they are all part of a common educational system. Some of the core philosophies, which distinguish a Montessori preschool from a traditional daycare, include:

Timeframe

A preschool Montessori loves energy and views every event as an opportunity to understand and teach. In a conventional daycare, the primary attention is put on childcare. The kids in a daycare center generally do not begin to learn critical concepts such as studying, writing, and mathematics until they start Kindergarten around age 5. Nevertheless, children start the learning cycle during infancy in a Montessori classroom, with the adoption of Montessori principles like self-directed practice and circle time, which promote self-control and focus.

Montessori ideology always emphasizes continuity over time. This explains why Montessori children can remain for several years with the same tutor, versus a regular daycare where the children are introduced to a different teacher every year. The extended time span with teachers allows Montessori children to bond on a deeper level with their teacher.

Most importantly, it will enable the teachers in their classroom to develop and implement a long term, individual learning plan for each child.

Versatility-Flexibility

Although the layout may be the emphasis of a conventional daycare classroom, a Montessori classroom promotes versatility. The caregivers in a daycare classroom will evaluate the activities that all children will do collectively daily and will provide a timeframe for completing each activity. On the other side, a Montessori teacher will stress each child's individual needs and allow the students to study and move at their own pace. Kids can travel about and explore comfortably in a Montessori classroom by participating in things that involve them and interacting with others. Every child can function and learn at their speed before they completely understand a topic. Other focus

Holistic Attitude:

While a typical daycare team is concerned with educating children and merely exposing them to simple instructional subjects, Montessori instructors are committed to creating well-educated, excellently rounded, and highly productive individuals. Through the holistic approach, Montessori children are cultivated by collaborating and working on pursuits as a group in developing social skills and steady life habits. The comprehensive solution often includes peer-to-peer mentoring, when older students are granted the ability to tutor younger students, cultivating qualities such as teamwork, altruism, and management.

Libertad:

The teaching system depends on instructor-led instruction for working in a typical daycare. Children are allowed to travel around the classroom openly in a Montessori nursery, discovering and participating in a range of tasks of their choosing. This liberty allows each student to learn in an engaging Montessori environment through hands-on communication. By resisting the repeated memorization of facts and definitions made inevitable by conventional education, the Montessori theory encourages children to cultivate a deep enjoyment of learning by enabling children to create their own.

2.3 The Working Principles of the Montessori Method

Montessori described learning and education as a complex process wherein children when put in an atmosphere

as per the "inner rules" of their lives, through their "voluntary labor." Kids, she said, aspire to attain practical freedom, instinctively and vigorously. An inherent desire, named by Montessori, a "divine impulse," activates the kid to self-practice to conduct growth-promoting acts that lead to further growth and enhanced independence. Autonomy for kids implies being able to do the stuff that keeps them ready for pressure from adults. To the kid, it requires being able to "do it all alone." Montessori understood that, on some occasions, adequate adult guidance is needed, which can be gradually reduced when children know how to do it by themselves. Determination, based on the right to be personality-active, is the basis for the virtues of persistence at a mission, patience in achieving something before it is completed well, and happiness at a job well performed — all-important attributes of an autonomous person with a degree of high confidence and self-esteem. Montessori is a teaching approach includes a rewording of a school concept.

She described a school as a structured environment where children can develop freely, within their own pace, unhindered by the unexpected unraveling of their natural abilities. The school's formal atmosphere allowed children to exercise and improve their perceptions and thoughts and gain greater freedom by using a graded sequence of self-correcting postmodern materials. Montessori said, "The school must allow the child's free, natural aspects if scientific philosophy is to be born in the school." Montessori modified the learning environment using her ideals of "the freedom of the learners in their serendipitous manifestations" and "liberty in an activity." She substituted the columns of immovable rigid desks in the traditional classroom with compact, child-sized chairs and tables, which the kids could push about. Montessori's classrooms featured a collection of open cupboards to store resources that could be easily reached by children. In her structured instructional setting, supervision (or management of the classroom) was reinterpreted to no further involve having children perched at their seats. This assumed the entire layout of the school, and the instructor's managerial style allowed pupils to regulate their internal behavior. Montessori said, "A space in which all children travel around in a pleasant, knowledgeable, and voluntary manner without doing any harsh or rude act will seem to be a rather well-controlled classroom indeed."

Child support

Love for the Child is the basic concept that underlies the whole Montessori system. Montessori claimed that infants

should be educated (in the early twentieth century, not standard practice). Respect for children is demonstrated by not disrupting their concentration. Regard is also demonstrated by giving students the freedom to make choices, do stuff for themselves, and learn for themselves. Teachers model consideration for all students and respectful resolution of conflicts, and must strive to observe without judgment.

The Absorption Meaning

Montessori teaching is focused on the idea that children are actively learning about the environment around them, only by living. Kinder are constantly absorbing information from their world through their senses. They make sense of it then because they are creatures of feeling.

Flexible timeframes

Montessori pedagogy believes that there are certain times during which children are more willing to learn those skills. These are regarded as sensitive periods, which last only as long as the child requires acquiring the skills. For each infant, the sequence in which sensitive periods exist (i.e., a sensitive period for writing) and the duration differ. Montessori teachers need to recognize sensitive periods of their students

by evaluation and provide the tools for children to thrive during this phase.

The environmental preparedness

The Montessori approach proposes that learners develop best in an environment designed to encourage them to do stuff independently. The learning environment should always be child-centered and should promote freedom for students to enjoy the resources of their choosing. Teachers can plan the learning atmosphere by providing support and activities accessible to children in an organized and autonomous manner.

Auto training

Auto schooling, or self-care, is the idea that children should teach themselves. This is one of the Montessori Method's most powerful principles. Montessori teachers provide children with the environment, inspiration, guidance, and encouragement to educate themselves.

Beauty

Environments at Montessori ought to be beautiful. Whether your school is in an old historic townhouse, in a strip-mall, or in your home's living room, the surroundings should offer a quick harmony. Uncluttered and well maintained, the

atmosphere will represent harmony and tranquility. The atmosphere will be motivating the learner to come in and work. This environment is clearly shown from the behavior of those employed there, both child and individual.

Nature and Truth

Montessori has a strong appreciation and admiration for nature. She presumed that we should use nature to motivate children. She perpetually recommended that Montessori teachers keep the kids out into nature, instead of keeping them restricted in the classroom. This is why organic fibers are favored in a structured environment. Real wood, reeds, teak, metal, cotton, and glass, are preferred over synthetic materials or plastics. It is here that real artifacts of children's scale come into action. Furnishings should be kid-sized, so the child is not reliant on the adult for his movement. Rakes, hoes, pitchers, utensils, shovels all should fit children's hands and height so that the work is made much easier, thus having correct use and execution of the project without frustration.

Montessori Curriculum

Functional Life Skills An essential aspect of the Montessori philosophy is to give children the freedom they need to develop themselves. Being free means, one has the power, the ability, to do what it takes to live. For infants, this independence means they would acquire the expertise and skills to conduct the activities of daily life, depending on their individual preparation and level of growth. The realistic life skills include a variety of practices intended to improve the confidence and self-reliance of the infant. The duties involve those things that are part of living in a home as a member of a family (setting the table, serving meals, preparing dishes, cleaning up after a meal); those necessary for personal cleanliness and grooming (washing your face and hands, brushing your teeth); and those needed to dress (buttoning your smocks and lacing and tying your shoes). Special didactic equipment — lacing and binding objects — offered children a chance to learn a particular talent. Included in the functional life skills were physical activities linked to physiological growth, such as muscle balance, driving, and respiratory skills. We managed to stick with a single talent through repeated exercises until they had perfected it. Through realistic social activities, the kids experience muscular coordination and gain knowledge to persevere in mastering a task.

Sensory Awareness

The sensory resources and exercises are meant to improve the sensory acuity and ability of the infant. Through utilizing specifically built instruments and products, children learn to arrange, identify and evaluate sensory experiences through observing, hearing, sensing, degusting, listening, and experiencing the physical properties of the items in the area. Sensory abilities include those related to sound and the ability to differentiate between tones; those related to sight and the ability to perceive and discern color, shadow, and hue; and those related to touch and the ability to sense strength, softness, stiffness, cold and fire. Specific didactic devices and products, such as tubes, tone rings, mounting plates, fabrics in various shades, and so on, were again used. The sensory education practices of Montessori have three predicted results: firstly, enhancing the sensory ability of children by using their forces of discrimination; secondly, enhancing the basic sensory functions of children; thirdly, increasing the preparation of children to carry out tasks that are more complex.

Visual Products

Montessori developed the products focused on children's scientific findings. She took each of the senses carefully and thought of how much she could help the kids understand and enhance their current interactions. Montessori concentrated on

"structures of artifacts exchanging certain attribute, including color, form, and dimension." She set out to plan the atmosphere, which gave a child the ability to engage with a material or a "product" quite explicitly.

Within Montessori, Sensorial is one of five main learning regions. The approach is to think about tactile as one way the child (aka "the Young Explorer") is trying to make sense of and learn his surroundings (akin to dialect and the alphanumeric characters). He classifies and generates balance by utilizing his senses of his comprehension, learning, and location in the universe. The main objective is this sense of order by isolating specific concepts in order to enable the child to learn simple information and make sense of this understanding within his context. Exercises are grouped into the following fields with an illustration of the material:

- Visual-Wide staircase

- Olfactory – Smelling Flasks Gustatory- To taste the Bottles

- Tactile-Flat and rugged frames

- Visual (Geometry)-Set of triangles

- Auditory-Valve tone

- Stereognosis – Mystery Pack

Every group of objects symbolizes the same efficiency but in various degrees. By removing or reducing certain distinctions, every content underlines one specific feature. Consequently, there is a normal yet incremental differentiation between the various items and, where appropriate, one that is set mathematically, like the Pink Tower and the metric method.

Language Skills

Montessori always said that language was the human force that transformed the raw world into society, as an instrument of collective human thinking. While all humans had the general power to learn and acquire language, the key element in identifying and separating a specific group of humans was a particular language. Kids learn the language along with all components of the environment. The acquisition of language, which Montessori differentiated from language instruction, is a natural product of the infant. For all children, language acquisition follows the same trends regardless of the specific language used in the culture of the child. All children go through a time where they can only say syllables, then entire sentences, and finally continue using vocabulary and grammar. Language learning started through sound and letter practice. Letters were cut out and placed on outlines of sandpaper, which could be tracked and pronounced phonetically by the youngsters. The children used the letters of a movable alphabet to compose words. Montessori believed the children exploded into writing and reading spontaneously. Arithmetic was demonstrated by the use of geometrically formed objects, the usage of rods of various lengths, and the arrangement of material amounts in counting boxes. Children traced numbers filled with sandpaper, while they studied the letters. More general physical, social and cultural skills were learned by individualized physical activities, mutual roles of caring for plants and animals, and universal regard for one's own job and others' work. Again, the children themselves formed an awareness of the larger world they existed in. As they provide structure to the sensory input they have acquired, they are becoming more aware that they need more Awareness regarding the wider environment they exist in.

2.4 Role of a Montessori Teacher and the Ideal Learning Environment

The educational approach of Montessori highlights children's improved cognitive capacity as they are empowered to make the right decisions. It started at the start of the 20th century to improve the education of children by helping them to help themselves. Today's curriculum for Montessori instructors is about learning this form of directing young minds. There are five features parents should picture for in educators when selecting a Montessori school for their kids.

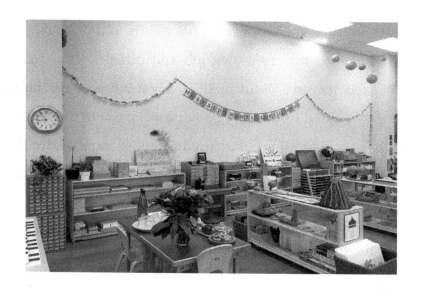

Sets a strong definition

Kids are fond of mimicking what they see and hear. This is a matter of the cycle of thinking. Montessori teachers set an example, facilitating children's understanding of how things work. These teachers are constant role models who set a great example in actions, interaction, and orderliness for students. The main form of a Montessori instructor is a role model is by viewing all children as people with great regard. A teacher at Montessori understands that a child's superpower is rampant curiosity. An instructor can more efficiently channel that interest into fruitful directions by carefully harnessing the power through compassion and acute observation. Therefore, children understand that their interest is important, valued, and a major part of their increasing self. We always know that teachers care about their needs, and will show them lessons that are enjoyable and interesting. That is how shared faith and reverence grows in a classroom at Montessori.

Taking special note

An instructor at Montessori utilizes methods that are somewhat distinct from what you, as a student, would be accustomed to in a typical classroom. Within a Montessori school, a blackboard has no line of chairs. A Montessori instructor quite seldom gets up and teaches for lengthy hours. Indeed, the Montessori ideology does set academic milestones for the advancement of a child, but the teaching itself is not done "top-down" through multiple quizzes, tests, and note-taking lessons, but rather from more of an organic "bottom-up" philosophy, taking indications from the children themselves for directing individualized education. One of the basics of the Montessori philosophy of education is that children advance at their own pace. Effective observers will provide the right information to lead students in the right way. In addition, when students are allowed to define what skills, knowledge, and move to the next level, they can sense more clearly. The significant distinction between the Montessori classroom environment versus a conventional nursery or daycare is the willingness to evaluate versus direct closely, instead of merely disciplining and taking control.

Takes a Connection

Even the toys in a Montessori school are different. Wisely made, bright, and eye-catching, such toys that appear to the neutral onlooker (and the child) as simplistic playthings, but each was built for learning. Lovely golden beads can be hung into wires to help older kids understand the decimal system. Multicolored cubes and orbs teach distinguishing abstract form and color. A button brace helps a child to focus on basic motor skills. As a bonus, if the buttons are done incorrectly, the kid can see immediately, so he can achieve independence by attempting to fix it himself. Throughout Montessori, learning, training educators are taught that their main function is to become the connection between the kids and their teaching resources. Teachers give lectures to the students creating the connection between a sense of wonder and child interaction. Parents taking into account which Montessori school to choose from must look for teachers who can interact well with children and where a child can easily access all of their classroom materials.

Flourishes on New Findings

People loving learning flourish on fresh findings. Educators who teach students to experience learning activities in an effective way are also keen to accept new things. Throughout the Montessori community, the children and teachers will benefit from each other. The inventor of this teaching approach (Dr. Maria Montessori) was an enthusiastic learner who, though dealing with a large array of youngsters, developed their own information base and studies. Montessori teachers not only understand from their students but also are also involved in ongoing professional growth. In addition, the American Montessori Society allows accredited teachers to take thirty to fifty hours of instruction every three to five years to continue keeping certificates, based on when the qualification was given. The key topics ranging from the syllabus, child development, managing classrooms, mental or psychological issues, and special education to skill training and educational strategy. These requirements are keeping Montessori teachers curious, engaged, and at the forefront of their profession.

Gains from Mistakes

If you have recently been to a school or college graduation, you may have observed that the topic of many a beginning speech focuses on the significance of "accepting failure." experts at the top of their disciplines understand that making wrong decisions is a given, and failure is inevitable. What an individual responds to failure is the distinguishing characteristic of some of the most successful and motivating individuals who have surmounted incredible obstacles by not letting failure dampen. The Montessori philosophy tends to revolve around supporting children not to be disheartened by errors, but rather to be emboldened, with polite guidance from the teachers, to correct them themselves. Guiding kids to understand that mistakes are happening and that blunders can be learning tools. Teachers trained in the Montessori learn what they say. Learning from errors will help them develop children's learning in the classroom.

Recognizes special education

These teachers must also finish at least a bachelor's degree before continuing to pursue Montessori training, aside from having specific qualities to be a Montessori teacher. The educational qualifications for becoming a teacher varies in each state and may differ based on the age group teaching.

Individuals with a college degree are qualified for an approved Montessori teaching program and can require one to 2 sequential summers to complete. It also requires a yearlong teaching internship before considering a teacher for a Montessori School.

Fosters Effort, Liberty, and Self-Confidence

Montessori education encourages children from an early age to provide self-reliance through educating teachers to be guided on the road to academic achievement for any child. An instructor at Montessori understands when to interfere and explain and when to stand back to let the child benefit about his own mistakes. A kid who knows how to belt, fasten buttons, and tie a knot by trial and error (and helpful guidance) will soon dress himself alone, confident of what he has accomplished. This emphasis on learning through experimentation, and taking errors in step, has domino-like implications. Pride of one's own achievements instills confidence. Trust promotes bravery and individuality. Independence triggers self-reliance. Such characteristics are impossible to "teach" from one's own experience through any approach other than trial-and-error. They are character qualities that will help children in the world no matter what they choose to do.

Fosters Creativity

If a kid is excited over something, there is no reason for him or her to be nagged, steered, or anxious to know more. Innovation is a source of imagination. Montessori instructors maintain detailed and personalized instructional strategies and expectations for growing students in the classroom, focused on close evaluation and regular record keeping. These strategies help to move the kids towards new milestones in educational, social, and growth. However, a teacher at Montessori does not force a child towards these milestones. Rather, he or she uses the child's own sense of wonder and innate, limitless creative thinking as the fuel for propelling the learner well past those deliverables. Back when more than a century ago, the Montessori ideology was still being developed, the methods of Maria Montessori were a dramatic shift from the standard systems of learning of the time. However, the philosophy of Maria Montessori was not a conceptual one, but an ideology formed out of years of empirical student observation in the classroom. Now it is regarded as a tried-and-true method of child development, and the schools of Montessori have spread throughout the world.

When you are contemplating your child to have a Montessori degree, engage in your innate curiosity. Read more about the theory of schooling, talk with fellow parents who have educated their own children, and experience an engaged classroom. Above all, take considerable time chatting with the teachers. They are the true heirs of Maria Montessori, proceeding to learn the joys, difficulties, and new adventures that their kids carry to the classroom on a daily basis.

The Ideal Montessori Instructor

The Montessori instructor, acting as a mentor and facilitator, provides a very well prepared Montessori setting and a prosperous and diligent experience intended to transfer learners from one task and stage to the next. The instructor from Montessori also stands back as the kids work, encouraging them to benefit from their own experiences and form an opinion. Rather than presenting solutions to students, the Montessori instructor tells them if they can fix the issue, consciously engage students with the learning process, and develop clear cognitive skills. For certain situations, rather than the tutor, children learn primarily from the environment, often from other students. Dr. Montessori claimed the instructor would concentrate on the infant as an individual rather than on the preparations for the everyday classes. The

Montessori instructor schedules regular courses because, for a growing child, she must be sensitive to shifts in the child's motivation, development, attitude, and actions.

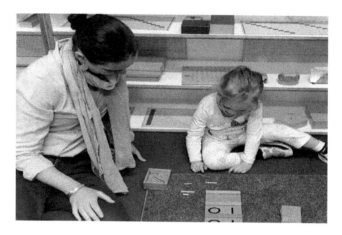

Sets a Good Example

Kids are fond of mimicking what they hear or see. It is a component of the method of learning. Montessori instructors usually lead by example, facilitating children's understanding of how things work. These teachers are continuous role models that set a great example in conduct, interaction, and tidiness for students. The main form of a Montessori instructor is a role model is by viewing all children as people with high regard. A teacher at Montessori recognizes that a child's superpower is widespread curiosity. An instructor can more successfully channel that interest into fruitful pathways by deliberately utilizing the capacity by compassion and acute observation. Therefore, children understand that their interest is essential, valued, and a significant part of their increasing self. They always know that educators care about their needs and will show them stuff that is enjoyable and interesting. That is how the relationship of trust develops in a classroom at Montessori.

Strengthening the Relationship

It has been found that good teaching has a clear connection with the quality of the relationships that occur between educators and particular children. In addition, mediocre teachers will be more effective than their technologically superior counterparts will if they can help cultivate their emotional connections with the students. Each relationship must be built separately, and the process does have a science or art. Ideally, any contact between both the child and Montessori educators will strengthen the fundamental emotional connection concurrently and understand the overall intent of the experience. There can be two aspects you might want to establish partnerships on. On the one hand, the teacher implements mechanisms and systems, which render daily interactions with each child possible. On the other hand, the teacher communicates spontaneously with and boy, with groups of kids, and with the class as a whole. It helps in the overall intensity of the community relationships with the teacher serving as a role model for a plurality of tender, growing relationships.

Teachers At Montessori Are Educated To Learn Like Scientists.

Members should be aware that teachers at Montessori are highly educated. In parallel to their college degrees, several have already accepted Montessori certificates. Montessori credential programs are rigorous and demanding; the equivalent of any college degree may be applied to them. Not only can these educational programs teach Montessori instructors how to utilize the advanced materials, but there are also comprehensive seminars on Montessori theory, infant growth, and arts incorporation. Montessori teachers do not depend solely on standardized tests when the needs come to assessments; they predict the outcome based on observation. They have brimming journals with proof of what their students learned, need more help, and are intrigued about. They actively log what they see kids focusing on, how the research is being done, and suggestions that they may have in expectation of the next steps of a project. Montessori teachers simply sit next to a child to determine exactly what they learn about a wide variety of areas of material.

Teachers at Montessori Foster Freedom

In a Montessori school, the instructor may interact individually with particular children or small classes, rather than having a teacher in the front of the school teaching any child the same lesson. When this occurs, the majority of the kids are safe to invest their time performing the job demanding on them. An instructor at Montessori is working hard to create systems that allow children to explore and trust themselves as learners. A significant portion of what a Montessori educator does is to deliberately prepare a developmentally appropriate classroom environment, invite children, and support them to work independently on their journey. This atmosphere is continually shifting in minute ways as the instructor considers the students' current and emerging needs.

Recording and Prep

Planning and record keeping reflect essential skills for becoming an excellent Montessori instructor. Plans will be made for a lengthy period as well as for one week, ensuring that all the children will get the lessons they need across a wide variety of subjects. It is also important to plan so that the children can be categorized correctly and according to their various standards, such as communities, special interests, and ability groups. Ultimately, preparation is what can allow an instructor to create appropriate decisions as the kids come up with different lesson demands. Efficient record keeping enables a teacher to have an ongoing allusion on which to base their preparation and from which to assess with frequent ease the advancement of each kid along with a wide range of sectors of development. Reliable records often come in handy for the next in line person to be the child's instructor because he/she would then be able to resume the child's school activities without contributing to any unwelcome interruptions. In this type of schooling, the lessons are best regarded as presentations. Dr. Montessori developed this framework with the entire idea of lessons on the hate of her parents. Rather, her inclination was to have a talk with the girls. Today, this experience has had a profound effect on the life of children and teachers through Montessori and has a strong influence on all takes place in the classroom. This also relates to how instructors at Montessori are educated in their different settings. Montessori demonstrations have a theory, and one of the most significant things is how the products in Montessori are put in the room. It is also quite important to take into account how and where to hold the presentation. Lastly, what would the presentation's closing theme be? Repetition will be promoted so that teachers can prepare with a range of strategies. Often, the activity you deliver as an instructor is merely replicated by the pupil. In other situations, the conclusion of a demonstration presents an opportunity to incorporate some new and exciting follow-up activities.

The Instructors At Montessori Are Also Named 'Guides.'

Although children have lots of flexibility in their educational activities at Montessori schools, Montessori is focused on the principle of 'independence inside boundaries.' This is the responsibility of the Montessori instructor to design certain boundaries with respect. Children depend on having developed a certain amount of support. This provides them with warmth, and healthy space to take chances and attempt new stuff. Teachers at Montessori establish such limits and then deliberately guide students to work inside them. What if your child in third grade is fond of reading but generally avoids mathematics? Their teacher at Montessori will seek to ensure that the mathematics is still done. This sometimes includes a polite conversation with a child on organizational skills, priorities, or goal setting. The instructor must also find a means of incorporating the child's desires into less favorable jobs. Sometimes, what it takes is a slight environmental improvement. Teachers from Montessori grant children independence, helping them find a path to progress in this world. Teachers at Montessori respect freedom, self-reliance, and inspiration inherent to them. They do admire mutual engagement, compassion, and power.

Chapter 3: Positive and Effective Parenting Strategies for Raising Disciplined Kids

In addition to being born harmless and good, each child comes into this world with its own different challenges. Our involvement as parents is to help the children face their particular problems. We can support our kids as parents but we cannot take away their particular struggles and issues. Through this perspective, we will be less concerned, rather than dwelling on improving them or fixing their problems. Trusting in more benefits both the parent and the boy. We should let our children be on their own, and concentrate more on having them develop in response to the difficulties of life. Children have a better ability to believe in themselves, their peers, and the uncertain future when peers react to their children from a more comfortable and confident position. Every child has a specific destiny of his or her own. Acceptance of this fact reassures parents, makes them cope, and does not assume blame for any child's problem. So much effort and money are lost on attempting to find out what we might have done differently or what our kids could have accomplished, instead of realizing that both kids have issues, problems, and obstacles. Our role as parents is to support our children to meet them and effectively deal with them. Know also that our kids have their own range of struggles and talents and there is nothing we can do to change who they are. In addition, we will ensure that we owe them the opportunity to become the greatest they can be.

Kids have their own range of struggles and talents so we cannot do much but change who they are. If we continue to believe something is wrong with our kids at tough moments, we have to come around and note that they are from heaven. We are great in their way of life and bring their own special problems. They need not only our compassion and help but their challenges as well. Their specific challenges to be conquered are in reality important to make them all that they can become. The challenges that they encounter will help them get the resources they need to grow their unique character.

The safe growth cycle ensures there will be hard times for any child. Kids can acquire such vital life skills as humility, deferred gratification, tolerance, teamwork, imagination, kindness, bravery, patience, self-correction, self-esteem, self-sufficiency, and self-direction by learning to recognize and tolerate the constraints imposed by their parents and the universe. For instance:

• Children cannot gain tolerance, or learn to postpone gratification because they want things to happen. Young

children cannot begin to apologize until anyone is around to accept.

• If everything around them is flawless, children cannot learn to tolerate their own flaws.

• Children cannot learn how to cooperate whenever everything goes their way.

• Children cannot strive to be imaginative because all is accomplished without them.

• Children cannot learn empathy and care without feeling pain and loss, too.

• If children face hardship, they cannot grow to be brave and hopeful.

• Unless children overcome obstacles to achieving something, they cannot feel self-esteem or happy pride.

• If the children undergo isolation or dismissal, they cannot establish self-sufficiency.

• Children are unable to develop perseverance and resilience when all is simple. Young children cannot learn to correct themselves until they encounter difficulty, mistake or error.

- Unless children have the opportunity to resist power and/or not be provided what they want, they cannot be self-directed. Challenge and increasing pain are not only unavoidable in a number of ways but also necessary. Our role as parents is not to shield our kids from the hardships of life but to help them successfully overcome and develop.

In chapters 3 and 4 of Toddler Discipline, you will develop new constructive coping strategies to help your kids adapt to the difficulties and failures of existence. If you still fix their issues, they do not consider their natural talents and strengths inside themselves. Challenges to life will arise in improving the kids in unusual ways and finding the best of them. There is a tremendous difficulty as a butterfly escapes from its protective bubble. If you break the cocoon open to save the battle for the new butterfly, it will soon die. It takes the struggle to get out building the wings. The butterflies can never travel without the battle but then perish. Similarly, specific types of struggle and a special kind of support is needed for our kids to gather strength and fly freely in this world. Every child needs a particular sort of love and support to surmount their unique challenges. Without such help, they will magnify and misrepresent their issues, even to the extent of psychiatric disorder and illegal activity. Our role as adults is to help our kids in different ways so that our kids get better and safer. If we intervene, make it even easier, we degrade kids, but if we make it too complicated, and do not support sufficiently, then we rob them of what they need to flourish. Children cannot do it by themselves. Without the support of their parents, a kid cannot grow up and learn all the skills for productive living.

3.1 Practicing Montessori from Day 1 & Creating an Ideal Montessori Environment at Home

Most parents are fascinated by the concept when it comes to integrating Montessori concepts at home, but they are not sure where to proceed. Still, it begins with a shift in attitude. As a parent, you must start by realizing that kids — including the smallest ones, know more than you will recognize. When you understand that, so you will make specific improvements in your house to set yourself and your infant up for success in Montessori.

We always expend time and resources proving the home for children but think their world as a whole until the child is not immensely grown-up but a toddler. A Montessori space's ideal is to be able to leave the room and be assured they are safe to play and discover by themselves. After all, "Help me do it by myself" is the Montessori motto. Put toys, books, and even clothes at their eye level. Get a little wooden table and benches, with some small open shelving (the method's cornerstone) and some artwork at their level so they can enjoy more!

Simplify

There is talk of the second open shelving; we immediately worry about having a disaster. However, Montessori's underlying philosophy is that it is in a peaceful and ordered setting where children grow best. Try getting rid of all the clutter while keeping just a couple of items out of the racks. You should pick up a decent chunk of toys and then toggle on fresh ones until they get sick of them. Essentially, it is a more streamlined strategy, which in effect makes the home tidier and the kid more active. Moreover, children tend to gravitate to just a few toys at a time, and never play with anything anyway! That will also help with unnecessary buying, as you are recycling what you already have instead of continually getting in new products.

Natural Should Be the Key

We all recognize the advantages of fresh air, play outdoors, and get dirty. However, the Montessori approach does not confine development to the outside. Bringing things inside is similarly worthwhile! It is an excellent idea to encourage children to gather and view such items as rocks, pinecones, or seashells. Frame the flowers they choose in your table area or using the slice of driftwood. Natural materials are a component in the design, too. Attempt to add various materials, such as cotton, fur, tons of wood, or bamboo. That often refers to toys – the Montessori approach is meant to reduce the amount of material that children interact with, preferring components that are more natural. This might be the toughest aspect, with the volume of technologies currently available. Only setting the aim of incorporating one wooden puzzle or shortening the screen time every day by a few minutes will make a difference.

Assemble the Setting

Montessori's vital values at home are "a location for all and all in its position." When you assign a location for it all, your child can soon know where it all goes. This is a valuable resource to encourage them to be accountable for their possessions and to wipe up messes that they are growing to create. The most crucial adjustment you would like to make to manage your world better is to make it more available to your kids.

To do so, parents are advised to:

- Place steps in both the kitchenette and bathroom to encourage them to clean their hands and help with the preparation of meals in the kitchen

- Place nutritious snacks low in your fridge or cupboard so that your kid can support himself.

- Hold clothes in small drawers or bins, and push the rope in the wardrobe down to the eye level so that your child can touch their garments.

- Keep drinks in comparatively tiny pitchers situated in the refrigerator on the bottom shelf, with cups that are child friendly and nearby. Enable them to support themselves when your child is hungry — make sure to have a sponge handy, which they can use to wipe up the little mess they make.

- Put toys, gaming tools, and craft supplies on bottom shelves where your child can quickly reach them, then split these toys into specific baskets, bins such that the products stay distinct, and are simple to locate without wading through loads of other gadgets.

Parents are often advised to change the toys and books for their children every few weeks in the Montessori Method. This is meant to maintain their attention alive and to avoid boredom. Any parents may consider this daunting, but the easiest approach to do it is to change the products on your shelves depending on the conditions and the real needs of your kid. Are they getting curious about pterosaurs? In addition, add a dinosaur box and a pair of age-appropriate textbooks on the shelf. Whichever topics your children are involved in, the aim is to promote creativity and creativeness.

Highlight Real-World Skills

Even young kids can pitch in around the living room. By training them to keep track of themselves at an early age and the environment surrounding them, you will eventually prepare the child to be a conscientious, willing person. It may suggest you will have to pause as a parent to take the time to show your child how to clean the table correctly during a meal or which cabinets to place their bottles in. Still, their brains are so permeable that it will not be long until they manage it individually.

Recognize to match age as well as ability with their chores. Relatively young children, for example, are perfectly able to learn water their plants, bring food for pets, sweep the table after lunch, and find up their toys. Older kids will integrate more complicated activities into their schedules, such as clearing the garbage, cooking meals, and simple home maintenance. Within your family, too, you might make them instruct the younger ones.

Create a Montessori Baby Environment

Kids are never too small for Montessori to start with. Martinez thinks it is better to view them, even when interacting with children, as whole entities from day one. "Maria Montessori spoke about the divine seed and how kids come into this world thinking and possessing all the knowledge they need to meet their needs, as well as being completely human," she asserts. It is everyone's duty to direct him or her in changing the future around him or her. Some things that can be done to integrate Montessori at home for your Baby:

• Choose the screen in monochrome. Forget all the chimes and buzzers of those over-stimulating smartphones. Martinez says an easy mobile in black and white is great for babies allured to better contrast images.

• Put tactile toys at close range. When kids grow older, Martinez advises placing Montessori infant toys within the range that they can move and even feel through their senses (for starters, objects through different textures).

• Hang the mirror on small. Putting some well-placed mirror at their point is fantastic for babies that get a kick out of to see their moves and finally realize that they are the picture they see.

• Think about that high chair. As long as your kid is sitting up safely, it is best to seek to have the balance at a table on a child-sized chair, Riordan suggests. From the moment they start solids, they can also exercise self-feeding.

• Insist on touch. The greatest infant toy is in contact with you and with the environment around them. These can involve listening to songs, enjoying them, or heading on nature walks.

• First position protection. Particularly when babies start running, you will follow the same childproofing precautions that you should elsewhere in a Montessori home: Anchor all large furniture, hold sharp items out of sight, cover electrical sockets, etc. When this is all, you will need to keep your kid out of dangerous places, using baby gates.

When your child ages and is more independent, offering the ability to travel and experience, their entire home is necessary. This means the entire baby proofing you did when they were babies will always be essential when they grow up — but you will want to change it when they evolve to compensate for their expanded independence and need for more space. As toilet training usually happens during the early childhood period, the Montessori activities may need to apply to the toilet, because the child may spend more time there. Including a stepladder, faucet connectors, and a light switch extender is necessary — all to train your toddler to be self-reliable when in the bathroom. The degree of play often changes as children mature. There is a variety of activities you should do to facilitate their curiosity about the environment around them like these three.

1. Hold Small Books and Toys

Put on low shelves a limited range of age-appropriate books and games-just no electronic items. Holding them in a little shelf would encourage your kid to occupy himself with something that catches his eye. Place through sort of product in another basket or bin, and they can start realizing anything has a proper location. Rotate their collection of toys and books every few weeks to keep it fresh and unique.

2. Hang Amazing Eye-Level Artwork

If it is a photo by one of the greats, or a painted picture your child or an older sibling created, introducing your kid to design and art is a great way to inspire their imagination.

3. Build real, seasonal trays

Each season put, together with a plate of items you have found outdoors to touch and explore your child. When you engage your child in gathering objects from your yard that can also become another learning and discovery moment. In addition, try to be sure there is nothing in the trays that might be a shock threat or render them uncomfortable if something winds up in their mouths.

If you are not sure where to proceed with a nature tray, take any of these seasonal ideas into account:

- Spring: Green leaves, mushrooms, assorted vegetables and bulbs, nuts, artificial eggs

- Summer: shells, tiny vessels, seeds, starfish, vegetables, herbs

- Fall: Gourds, berries, seeds, acorns, dry grain, fall papers, actual or artificial mummies

- Winter: snowflakes, leafy trees, snow globe, nature landscape photos

Creating a Pre-School Montessori Atmosphere At Home

From the time your kid becomes a preschooler (and even beyond), they are much more aware of becoming independent — and this should be mirrored in their community. "Three- to five-year-olds often practice all of the stuff they did while they were young, albeit in a more relaxed and focused manner," Martinez observes. Take into account all of the above suggestions for younger ages as you further extend your preschoolers' mobility inside the family.

• Montessori mattress. For preschoolers, a lower-to-the-ground mattress is often the better choice, but Martinez says her two children are in a small Ikea bunk bed to optimize their room.

• Hold clothes within sight. Whether you are using drawers, cabinets, or bins, the child's garments should be held at their level and make it easy for them to choose garments and attire themselves. • Keep your kid in mind on the fridge. Robinson recommends having lunch or snack items in the refrigerator and storeroom lower shelves so that the children can feed themselves. Retain the screens. Dr. Montessori did not want to think about seeing infants overwhelmed with screen time, so it is something that parents have to deal with today.

Robinson suggests they do not consider exposing children to computers in the Montessori schools before primary school and suggest that families do the same.

Sorting Out Issues at The Peace Table

When children need help solving problems, directing them to the table of peace can help them find phrases to settle their differences.

Children fall out with parents or peers from time to time — it can be over something as easy as playing with a doll or over a bigger problem like friendships. Often they hit the stage that they are too frustrated to negotiate with each other. This is where the peace table tends to come in, providing a place for the kids to cool off as they follow a procedure that will stop the argument in their tracks. The peace table is usually a table with two chairs, a bell, and a flower ornament symbolizing peace, maybe a rose, an olive twig, or a dove. Two chairs together are perfect, or a rug in the corner of a house, or even a particular place on the stairs if you're short of space. As children are used to the practice they may agree to go to the peace table without being spurred; on certain occasions, a parent or older sibling might see a conflict emerging and recommend that the members seek to fix their dilemma at the peace table. A certain protocol ensues while at the table. The child who feels especially wrong puts one hand on the table and the other hand on the head, signaling from the core that she is telling the facts. She then looks at the other child, speaks her name, and explains how she feels about what has happened and how she wants to settle the disagreement. The second child then gets a turn and the conversation, before an understanding is found, begins. When the children themselves cannot do that, they will require a mediator — may be an older sibling or a relative. If the issue is so much involved, they can call for a family conference, where the whole family listens to the tale from both sides. What children learn from the peace table is that their point of view will be heard regardless of their size, age, or position within the family and they can expect fair treatment. The central insight they obtain from these exercises is that to preserve a harmonious, peaceful environment at home, disputes must be concluded frankly and with goodwill.

3.2 Understanding Positive Parenting

In any stage of existence, several people become guardians. So while many of us aspire to be better parents, the seemingly relentless complexities of parenthood can often annoy so frustrate us. As both the parents of infants and teenagers will testify, these difficulties are apparent at all stages of development.

Soft Parenting

Most of the parents give up rough parenting. They acknowledge the importance of listening but do not understand how important it is to be the leader. By listening, and then placing the child, they try to avoid the resistance of their children. They listen, but instead, they give in to the reluctance of their child to keep the child comfortable. They cannot stand watching their kids sad and so they make whatever compromises they can to satisfy. This soft-love parenting brand is not working and has made many parents suspicious of positive parenting's new nurturing skills. Positive-parenting skills are fortunately working immediately. They are working both in the short term and in the end.

The weakness of parenting with unconditional touch leaves other parents wary of positive-parenting strategies. Soft-loving parents sometimes give in to the desires and wishes of their child, because they simply do not know what else to do to stop the tantrum. They try to do what they did when they grew up but they do not know any other way that operates.

They realize that it does not work to stretch and blame but they do not realize what it is. They mistakenly deliver the message by indulging their children that have fits or being challenging is a good way to get what you want. Soft-love parenting tries to make the child please and please.

Soft-loving parents will do their utmost to avoid a confrontation with their child. They do not know what to do when the children oppose a request and create new ways of avoiding resistance from their children and motivating collaboration. We are sending the impression that refusing is good, but they are not ensuring that they are the leader. To avoid resistance from a child, many parents are even taught to always give a child a choice by well-meaning experts. Giving choices will diminish resistance, but it will not create cooperation. It is another way to transfer so much authority to a kid and to undermine the boss's control.

A kid does not require options before the age of nine. Too many opportunities drive a child to develop so fast. So many options are perhaps the main causes of tension for adults today. Ask a young child straight away what she needs is placing so much strain on the girl. Asking kids constantly, what they want, or how they feel weakens the willingness of a parent to maintain control. Greater independence and transparency can cause more fear before we are able. Kids under nine are not equipped for it. They need strong parents who know what best for them, but who are also opens to listening to their resistance and discovering their wishes and wants. After the wishes and desires of a child have been discovered, parents can then try to change their direction or hold firm. The adult is still in control, though. The concept is similar to our form of justice. Once a trial is resolved, it cannot be revived unless additional evidence exists.

Similarly, although a kid may refuse, it does not imply that from his or her point of view the adult should budge. If the parent gets new insight through listening to the child, reconsidering what is to be done is fine. Parents can change their minds, not because they are afraid of opposition, but because they find new information that has changed their point of view. Parents will not amend their appeal, nor does the legal system, until additional evidence is available. Children need powerful parents who know what is best; no more choices are needed. Parents with soft love do not realize that resistance is essential need children have. Children ought to check the boundaries to make sure it is very relevant to what you want them to do. Otherwise, they have things they deem more important to do. Just as children need approval to resist and test their limits, they need a strong parent to listen to and then decide what is best. Strong parents still make a choice, since they are the supervisor. Children are not willing to self-employ. They need a boss. They start to self-destruct, without a boss. Soft, permissive parenting minimizes short-term opposition, however, weakens the ability of the children to participate. Girls tend to lack confidence because of hard parenting, whilst boys lack compassion. Girls tend to have low self-esteem because of soft upbringing and offer too much later in life, whereas boys are hyperactive and lose confidence and discipline.

Using positive-parenting techniques involves feeling opposition from your kid and then choosing what is right. Deciding what is best does not mean you are not deviating from the original position. When the kids are more conscious of what they need and desire, they also become better negotiators and are willing to convince you to change your mind. There is a vast difference between giving in to the feelings or wishes of your child and changing what you think it ought to do. Parents are the supervisor, but their order or point of view need not necessarily be adhered to rigidly. Listening to the opposition of a child involves knowing what he or she thinks and desires, then determining what is possible and then persisting. It is great to start telling the nine-year-old and older kids what they specifically believe, like, expect or need. Then it is at the age of twelve to fourteen when it is time to start telling teenagers what they think. The advancement of abstract thinking at puberty is a sign of the ability of children to start making their own decisions. The way we communicate with our children must always be age-appropriate. Children need to get a clear message at every age that making mistakes is okay. The best way to teach this is through learning from your own mistakes. The reality is parents are not always correct and they do not always know what is best. If they recognize and note the opposition of their child, they will know better. If parents shift their viewpoint, it will be because they have noticed something and agree that a shift is right. They do not adjust their perspective to mitigate the resistance of a boy. Placing the kids to reduce resistance just paves the way for greater potential resistance

However, there is good news — numerous resources and approaches, including this book, is backed by studies and is now conveniently accessible to parents. This chapter of the book offers a variety of knowledge about typical parental difficulties (i.e., bedtime conflicts, picky eating, outbursts, attitude concerns, risk-taking, etc.); and also the various life experiences that are actually part of the learning process (i.e., beginning kindergarten, being polite, having friends, becoming responsible, having healthy decisions, etc.). With its emphasis on satisfaction, optimism, and healthy growth of the youth, the area of positive psychology is especially important to successful parenting discussions. In addition, if you are a mom hoping to avoid future problems, or you are tearing your skin out already — you have found the right book.

Positive parenting is a collection of parenting techniques inspired by the work of Alfred Adler and Rudolf Dreikurs, the Viennese psychiatrists. Dr. Jane Nelsen Ed. D. in recent years, I on her famous series of books, refined and advocated this method and brought important positive parenting techniques well known. Constructive parenting strategies promote shared understanding and make use of constructive corrective guidance. The positive discipline relies on educating (future behavior), rather than prosecuting (past misconduct). Studies consistently show that the use of positive discipline results in better actions, personal healing, academic performance, and mental health outcomes for children.

A common trend in the successful parenting discourse is that multiple effective youth results equate a moist and strong parenting style. This style is called 'authoritative' and is conceived as a parenting model that combines a fine blend of the following parenting attributes assertive, but not disruptive, demanding, but flexible; disciplinary but not punitive (The year 1911, Baumrind). A developmental parenting style is often assumed to promote good child results within an authoritarian parenting style (Roggman et al., 2008). Along with therapist Rudolf Dreikers, Adler concluded that children should be handled with dignity but also urged parents to stop spoiling and coddling them, because these parenting techniques often produce more emotional and behavioral problems — feelings of superiority, self-centeredness, loss of empathy, etc. While some may find these two beliefs contradictory, in brief, positive parenting actually encourages parents to be empathetic and firm. It was this concept that led Jane Nelsen, Ed. D. - that parents should be both respectful and firm. Create the Constructive Training approach practiced by parents around the globe. The revolutionary concept has become the foundation of successful parenting. Many optimistic parenting experts will rely on the same three concepts from this paragraph.

Assumption 1: The primary objective of a child is to attain belonging and importance

Once a kid is clothed, fed, as well as housed, his next two withdrawal symptoms are for these basic needs: belonging and feeling significant. To belong is to feel needed and linked. Human beings are social beings — we long to become a part of something greater than us. Belonging to a kid involves feeling deeply linked to the significant characters in the story and feeling positive about how he works in your family. When major life shifts happen, a child's sense of self sometimes is rocked - like when a new baby comes or parents' divorce. These kinds of improvements can contribute to regressive habits, so once you realize where certain patterns come from, you can successfully fix them.

What is the significance? It can be defined is the sensation of being competent and desired. A child wants to realize that by making positive feedback he will create a difference inside a family. Moreover, he has to be able to exert his own personal power over his world. Every human being (child and adult) has an intrinsic need for control and the free will to choose whether to wield it. If children are unable to exercise their free will in a positive way, they will use pessimistic ways to gain control of what they want: unwilling to collaborate, speaking directly, doing the contrary of what you ask, pushing your buttons purposely.

Assumption 2: All behavior is target driven

Remember that your teen refused to do his homework? In addition, your preference for 5th graders not to listen? How about your awesome mealtime fight with 3-year-olds? Whether your child can express the ambition behind their selection (and do not worry, most cannot), we know from Adler's work that misconduct is simply an effort by a child to attain belonging and meaning. Once we recognize that misbehaviors are symptoms and not the real problem, we can tackle the root cause in a way that ultimately results. It is not that your originally used parenting techniques are technically wrong; they are not addressing the root of the problem. They simply put a sticking plaster on the exterior of a deeply rooted problem that can always hemorrhage.

Assumption 3: A Misbehaving Child Is a dissuaded Child

Just think about it for a second.

- A child who misbehaved is not a bad child.

- A kid who misbehaved is not an uncontrollable boy.

- A child with misbehavior is not a mean child.

- A kid who is misbehaving is not a stubborn boy.

- A child who is misbehaving is simply disheartened.

According to Alfred Adler, 'discouraged' in this sense specifically means the desires of the infant for identity and significance are not being fulfilled. It is his way of describing, "I don't feel like I belong or I don't have enough power over my own life, and this is the only method I can demonstrate to you how I feel." When your child is misbehaving, see it as a cry for help — understanding that something is not right for them. Sadly, for youngsters, because they do not find a constructive way to satisfy their emotional needs, they can do so simply by showing aggressive behaviors. If the feelings of a child's disparagement continue for a longer length of time, you will see that they repeat common inappropriate behaviors. Over time, the child will start believing that their misbehaviors will provide them the focus they desire or give them the feeling of control they are looking for. However, as we change our perspective to interpret the misbehavior as and Indication that something is wrong instead of treating it as a weakness on our part or a flaw of our infant, we can see behavior progress almost instantaneously.

Developmental area of parenting is a supportive parenting approach that facilitates successful infant development through:

- the delivery of empathy (i.e., by encouraging gestures of love for the infant)

- sensitivity (i.e., through taking note of the signals of the child)

- motivation (i.e., through promoting the strengths and desires of the child)

- instruction (i.e., through utilizing play and interaction to enhance the cognitive development of the child)

Developmental parenting evidently expresses several similarities with authoritative parenting styles, and both constitute positive approaches to parenting. The Council of Europe's Committee of Ministers (in the year 2006) defined similarly positive parenting as "caring, encouraging, non-violent" and "providing recognition and encouragement that involves setting limits to allow the child's full development" (in Rodrigo et al., 2012, p. 4). Combined with the constructive research on parenting, these concepts indicate the following about successful parenting:

- It includes guidance

- It involves taking the lead

- It's Careful

- It is Non-violent

- It provides free, daily contact

- It induces love

- It's Nourishing

- It is receptive to the needs of the child

- It shows Empathy for Feelings of the Child

- It serves the Child's Best Interests

- It provides Emotional Protection

- It gives energy to the emotions

- It offers Unconditional Affection

- It respects the developmental stage of children

- It establishes frontiers

Get To the Root of Your Conduct

Good parenting specialists around the globe will rely on this: There is often something that motivates the bad or destructive actions of an infant. There is always an explanation of why kids misbehave even if the parents that believe the cause is dumb. The child is reasonable, and that is why they behave like that. If parents can tackle the cause immediately, even if they do not get what they want, they would feel their needs are being recognized. Then they can move on without having to misbehave.

They could still be irritable, but once they feel understood, they do not need to act out. In the first instance, understanding the purpose behind can also help families stop them. So that meltdown over the blue plate? This was not a spontaneous show of bad judgment-it was fundamentally inspired by something about your kid. Whether it was a lack of skill in handling his significant feelings, a willingness to get your focus, or a penalty kill to affirm his free will – there has to be a reason for the behavior. (Even though he doesn't know it – because he doesn't! much of the time) The point to note that the actual action that actually the effect. Our job as parents is to find out what underneath the challenging activity really is.

It would make matters much simpler and easier if your kid could simply say, "Mummy, whenever I have you all to myself, I would very much like some one-on-one focus from you. Is there a chance we could do that tonight? "Yet that is an unrealistic concept we both realize. However, kids press our buttons then as a way to get our focus, although harmful. Also, because reality is, if a kid does not continue receiving our attention in beneficial ways (when they would not have to beg for it or ask for it), they will look for ways to get any recognition they can, even bad ones. Just imagine yourself as an investigator. When a child starts acting out, ask yourself, "What is this kid trying to achieve through his actions? "If he had the verbal abilities and emotional awareness, "What would he attempt to tell me about this behavior? Once the root cause of the issue is identified, you could become a more Flexible parent and prevent the tantrums from happening initially. Imagine, for instance, that you have to take an important phone call, but while you are on the phone, your kids decide it is a good reason to start a wrestling match. As you are already striving to sound interested in phone talk, you are offering your kids the look "if you're not stopping this right now, I'm going to lose it when I'm finished" – just for no reason. You start with the non-verbal shushing when fleeing from one space to the next in pursuit of quietness. However, the grappling match continues to overtake you. It is getting exhausting. So by the end of the line, you feel like you have just been running 5 miles. The primary objective behind such a wrestling match was most probable to get your recognition and push your buttons – which just happened to take the minute you got on the device. They knew that you were stranded on the phone and that you will be unable to take action, so it was the ideal time to act up and get your interest in negative ways. Using this as a learning tool and for the next time, you decide to talk over the phone.

Timeout

You have to start taking yourself on a timeout when required. It is unavoidable that parents are sometimes obviously exhausted and enraged by the unruly activities of children. However, this is the completely accurate moment of do-as-I-say-AND-as-I-do if you really can calm down and talk in a courteous and firm manner.

Think about it as well, when something does not go the way for your child, would you like them to explode, or would you like them to be capable of controlling their own emotions and remain civil? When you feel you are just about to abandon it all, show your daughter that because you are upset, you need a particular time of it alone. Give a timeline when you are going to come back and then go to some other room. Stepping back not only stops the fight for control but also enables you time to cool down and remember your goal of disciplining (which should be teaching, not winning in a conflict). While you are there, take deep breaths and take a few seconds to clear your mind. The timeout strategy often allows you some flexibility and a bit of breathing space to talk about how to cope with the issue. You are renewed as you return and able to take up the mission again. It has been shown that mindfulness exercise helps to reduce stress in such situations and promotes careful parenting.

Stick To It

While mothers know the significance of consistency intellectually, the reality is, life happens- the school is canceled, plans are changed, last-minute adjustments are made to the calendar. While we cannot all monitor life happens, much of the time, it is easier to have regular habits, schedules, and goals in your house. What is your morning routine like? If your kids are poised to make their blankets, brush their teeth, and dress before eating breakfast, keep this routine going every day. Retain the same weekends and holiday's routine. That way, you do not have to encounter Do you maintain the "policies of firm technology?" The Monday morning backslide! What happens if your children do not agree with technology laws in your family? To be the good parent you aspire to be, it is important that the laws of technology are explicitly articulated and that children recognize the repercussions if such rules are breached. If kids refuse to or "forget" to switch off the video game when the time is up, follow with the discussed earlier consequence every time. Children are far less eager to force the limits when parents are compliant with the rules.

Discipline, Do Not Criticize

The focus on discipline over punishment is one of the greatest key differences among positive parenting techniques and other methods of parentage. Discipline implies "training by discipline and practice," while punishing implies "inflicting punishment for (offense, blame, etc.)" or "strictly or badly treated." By educating our children on the best ways to act without the use of methods of discipline such as guilt, embarrassment, and discomfort, we train them and encourage them to be capable and effective young adults.

As per Positive Discipline: Dr. Jane Nelsen's First Three Years, punitive penalty comprises four Rs that do not help a child learn – Rebellion, Resentment, Retreat, and Revenge. Often punishment cannot stop bad behavior, and it does not teach good ones either. A beneficial, non-punitive reaction is much smarter for resolving and attempting to engage the over-stimulated child in developing basic behavior. One such reaction is to use positive timeout, or sometimes a time-in is called. A positive timeout is different from a conventional timeout that many parents use because it is not punitive. It is not fine. The child is excluded from the motivating environment that provides or aggravates misconduct and placed in a place where it can cool off and feel secure. The full term of timeout is Time off from Constructive Thinking, discovered while he was parenting his own children by a developmental scientist, Arthur Staats. The aim is to isolate the kid from the area where the troublesome activity happens in order to prevent any strengthening. The child eventually settles down and learns to lessen or halt unwanted behavior.

Unfortunately, it is misused as a form of punishment by many parents. During the timeout, they separate and limit the activity of the infant, then introduce a supplementary discipline by chastising and then lecturing the infant. Here are the key points to make proper use of timeout:

- Assert your expectations (dog not hit) and repercussion (timeout) clearly in advance. The kid needs to know that his or her own action can choose the consequence. This method lets them improve critical reasoning and make decisions.

- If the kid wants to do the inappropriate behavior, advise them gently and then escort them to a private, secure spot. Do not call them names, scold, look hateful, or be mean. That is, when you are using a timeout, be kind and firm.

If that makes her settle down, let your child watch cartoons, or wander about. Perhaps you should curl up and cuddle with them while they are frustrated. Know the constructive attitude to parents is not a threat. After that, describe (not debate) why their prior action was unacceptable and help them to come up with a decent response when they feel like acting out next time.

Making It an Opportunity for Learning

When children are mature enough to think (greater than three), every incident of misbehavior may be transformed into an important lesson in life. For example, what teaching moment is it to break a toy? Which indicates the kid will no longer interact with it. If the child did not like the toy, he should have just provided it to a friend or donated it for other children to enjoy. If they decided to break a toy out of anger, help them identify other outlets, such as kicking a pillow, to release the rage. It is always a perfect way to teach them words to describe their emotions instead of acting out ("I 'm mad because ..."). Around the same time, you are helping your child improve their cognitive abilities, which can greatly

decrease temperature tantrums.

3.3 Golden Rules to Discipline Your Child

The basic manners are one type of education for which infants are ready. No, not the technique of utilizing social introductions, or which fork. It is time to set the foundations to help your child develop into a respectful, considerate adult. How do you do that? Be kind about yourself. It is simple but obvious: Little potatoes have big eyes. They observe everything you do and they learn several ideas about how to conduct themselves by observation. Though infants are famously self-centered, by your example they begin to learn to take into account the feelings of others. Let them see you tell them "Hi," "Can I? "And" Sorry.

Tell your child how acts have repercussions about how they make people feel. For example, you could say after an argument, "See how sad it's when you reach Amber? Can you think of a way to make her feel better? "Use this method also to illustrate the impact of healthy behaviors. "Does it not make you sound good when you get a kiss from Aunt Sue? "Let's send Mrs. Smith some of the flowers we've selected, and see if it makes her happy." Please teach and thank you. Your child will probably pick up thank you naturally, and at a surprisingly early age, if he hears you use it every time he gives you things. With yes, you will have to ask it yourself at first, or promptly: "Can you type 'please'? "In addition, you are likely to keep prompting the kindergarten far past. Yet your patience will inevitably be rewarded and the habit will become entrenched. Just when to run it. Bear in mind the stage of your child's growth. An 18-month-old is unlikely to grasp the notion of sharing his toys with a stranger, so do not assume him a good host such is the way. In addition, when a kid is sleepy, starving, or sick, do not foresee any civility of any sort.

Discipline

The term 'discipline' often has a different meaning, which is purely punitive. In fact, 'discipline' is defined, however, as 'training that fixes changes or perfects the mental abilities or moralities of the character.

This description is instructive because it tells us that we are not disciplinarians as parents but more like teachers. In addition, as educators of our children, our point is to demonstrate to them respectful behavioral choices and to strengthen behavioral change in a positive way. Once again, positive discipline harks back to authoritative parenting, because it should be assessed in a manner that is both firm and affectionate. Positive discipline is most importantly never abusive, violent, or dismissive; it is not punitive. Physical punishment (i.e., slap across the face) is inefficient for long-term behavior change and has several negative effects on kids (Gershoff, 2013). The goal of constructive discipline, in reality, is to "teach and prepare." Punishment (pain/purpose damage inflicted) is needless and counter-productive" (2006, Kersey)

Nelsen (2006) describes a feeling of belonging as all people's main goal; a goal that is not accomplished through punishment. She shows the different negative effects of punishment on children (e.g., "the four R's") as resentment towards family members; revenge that can be arranged to get back to parents; rebellion against parents, including through much more increased attitudes; and retreat, which may require becoming devious and/or losing self-esteem (Nelsen, 2006). She offers the following five factors for positive discipline:

- Is Firm and Soft

- Promotes the sense of belonging and importance of a child

- Is not temporary, lasts much longer (note: punishment can have an instant effect but it's short-lived)

- Teach appreciable social and life skills (i.e. problem-solving skills, social skills, self-relieving, etc.)

- Allows learners to develop a feeling of being capable individuals

Family Ground Rules

Usually, there are far too many rules in some families when all that is required are some general steps that facilitate what we hope and expect from all members of the human race. There is no need to be tough or creative in making something about governing every element of the lives of your children. Agree on basic rules for your family and get them made d own and shown where both parents are allowed to refer to them. Teach your kid how to do the correct thing, instead of dwelling on his errors. There are normally just these few basic rules in the Montessori-inspired home (an ideal growing environment for your child):

• Treat others with respect.

• If you are using anything, put it right back when you are done.

• When something breaks or spills out, clean it.

• Say the truth and do not be afraid to confess when you make mistakes. You will keep the family ground rules plain in mind. Explain these positively, not as restrictions. Rather than saying: "don't go there!" Your kid will be asked what laws he will follow. Teach him how to implement them as if you were educating everyday life skills at any lesson.

Model a certain behavioral pattern you try to promote in your child. Try consciously to draw your child to do something appropriate and reinforce and appreciate even the tiny steps in that direction he is taking. Do not wait until a new skill has been mastered-encourage him all along the way. There are many ways you may do other than chastise, intimidate, or discipline while your child is violating a ground law. You can redirect him by suggesting a more suitable choice. You can remind him of ground rule, and ask him to stop politely but firmly. If the situation is not emotionally charged (such that, if you are not personally aggravated), the basic lesson about how to manage such situations can be re-read.

Be consistent. If you find you cannot get yourself to reinforce a rule repeatedly, that should not be a ground-rule. There are a few good rules that are much better than dozens, which are often ignored. Cut the word "no" eventually, each child will say stubbornly: "No, I don't want to!" This is a struggle for power that begins in the infancy years and often goes on during early adolescence. Numerous people call the "terrible twos" the toddler stage, but they do not have to be — not with two-year-olds or older children. Power struggles take place in situations where adults and children are determined to take their path, and no party is willing to go back down. Below, each one feels threatened and frustrated. The parents feel their children are challenging their authority directly. Children in situations like this usually feel powerless and try to assert their independence in their parental figure and establish more of a power balance.

Effective practice needs an initial upfront investment. However, in the end, your initial investments would get great behavioral payoffs. Below are ways to get you going when it comes to learning how to successfully motivate your child to obtain long-term results:

Fulfill Your Child's Attention Needs

Children need treatment, pure and basic. When we do not hold this "feedback box" full of constructive publicity, kids may be searching for whatever feedback they might find –

also negative. They will push our knobs with destructive emotions because even negative attention in the attention bucket is a "deposit" to the child.

However this doesn't mean you have to be on the side of your child 24/7 – just having taken a few minutes a day with your child to spend one-on-one, nuisance-free, and doing something they would like to do, will reap enormous benefits in their behavior. Take 15 minutes with each child once or twice a day, and play a game they have selected or read their favorite novel. Let the handset turn to voicemail. Do not answer the email. Just let dishes remain in the lavatory. When you fill the attention baskets for your kids strongly and constructively, your children will become more collaborative and less inclined to attract attention in a bad manner.

Life is busy for everybody, so having extra time in the day can at first be overwhelming, but think of that as an investment in your friendship with your kids so enhancing their behavior. In the first place, trying to give them what they need to avoid impoverished behavior patterns can have a huge role when it comes to realizing how to raise your child.

Take the Opportunity to Practice

It is important to keep in mind the root meaning of the word as you think about how to discipline your child – learn, advise, guide, instruct. The correct method to discipline your child is by teaching her the right behavior or response, to help her make better choices.

Role-playing is an ideal means of achieving so. For example, if your child has problems sharing and this outcome in whacking another child instead of whisking her aside to time-out, ease the tension, and show her the right way to react.

"When you're finished, I'd really like to play with the tractor." Alternatively, if your kid has a tantrum because they are hungry, show them the right words to use, "I'd like a snack, please." In addition, here is the fun part – swap roles, imagine that you are the kid, and let your little one steer you via better option. In addition, recognize this will take on accuracy and repetition like anything else. Do not expect a proper response from your child after one round of role-playing. Practice however makes progress and advancement make your home more peaceful.

Set the Goal and Hold On To It

Given the hectic schedule that plagues households nowadays, staying compliant with everyday routines can be challenging. Yet the fact is that while kids have the stability they succeed and learn their limits. If goals are expressed explicitly in advance, the children have a context through which to function.

This does not imply that you need to go crazy with hundreds of laws, but just concentrate on what is most important to your children. Be particular about the basic rules and what would be the consequences if someone violates the rules – make sure that everyone in the house realizes the results before time and that the discipline is linked with the misbehavior. When he fails to conform to the time limits for technology, he loses his technology rights for the following day or week (depending on age). However, it is not relevant to making her clean the basement because she did not do her homework, and therefore is not a suitable consequence. So be truthful above all. Respond with the agreed-upon outcome any time children break the rules.

Replacing Punishment

Positive Discipline has no spot for punishment. Why? For what? Thousands of research studies have shown that punishment is not the most effective way of teaching positive results. Rather it upsets, it makes others feel terrible, and it makes use of fear as a motivator.

Then why should many parents use approaches that are coercive or abusive? Just. Simple. They believe it works and that instead of allowing their children to "go away with" misbehavior they are "doing something." Punishment is a release for their wrath and frustration. Others use punishment for being conditioned by experiences and lacking the knowledge and skills to use different methods. They agree that the safest way for children to know is spanking, punishing, or take rights away. They are persuaded that they deserve to pay for schooling.

Often parents use punishment because it gives them a feeling of being in control — especially when punishment prevents the issue shortly. They do not want to be permissive so they believe punishment is the only alternative. When these parents stand back to take an unbiased glance, they find they are abusing time to again for the same behavior. That is a clear sign that retribution is not effective in the long term. If this definition suits you, you would be glad to know that you will learn other compassionate forms of training in this book, which are neither coercive nor permissive. Many parents also use retribution, because the human instinct is to take the least resistance course. The old pattern is almost difficult to shake unless you have anything new to substitute it. Always try to stop smoking, or lose weight. A void is abhorred by humans' consciousness. Starting something different is better than removing anything you are used to, then replacing it with nothing. A very small amount of constructive learning can be done with anger and negative energy output. Sometimes, when the kids believe you are upset at them, they act worse. Discipline, in order to be efficient, must be reasonable and caring (at the same time, compassionate and firm). Although it is good to reassure your kid that you are upset about a specific action, shouting out a penalty in frustration is counter-productive. There is a significant gap between the two.

Throughout this book, we will share many choices of ways to replace punishment with opportunities to learn with respect. Positive Discipline methods focus on teaching kids that their behavior affects others and that an adult will help them stop if they hurt others. They also understand that feeling a certain way about a situation is not an excuse to avoid addressing situational needs. Here are only a few instances.

• Your kid sprinkles his juice. Punitive parents would start shouting, hit, or angrily take away the juice, but you will grab a cloth for yourself and one for your child and say, "Clean it up together."

• You fail to do a job. Punitive parents take the privilege away, and the chore is still undone. Yet you are seeing your kid, having eye contact, and suggesting, "Time to finish the job." When your child responds, "Tomorrow," you are thinking, "I want you to honor your commitment. This is the moment to perform the job.'

• A tiny kid strikes you. Punitive parents struck back, yelled, or threatened. You take the hand of your child and cover yourself softly with it saying, "Cover, pat, pat. Be soft on that.

• The kid interacts with the dog very harshly. Punitive parents grumble, complain, nag, taunt, and scream. You split the two and inform them both, "When you are able to play more softly you two can try again later."

• Your child plays with a toy, roughly. Punitive parents use emotional manipulation, saying, "You're such a child. You are egotistical. You are too tiresome, "thinking the threats would inspire their kids to do better. Yet you are taking the set, placing it in a secure position, and saying, "Let me know when you're able to try again and play more softly." "I'm ready" and continues to play roughly, put away the toy and say, "When I'm ready to try again I'll let you know."

You will find that parents who use Constructive Reinforcement do not neglect problems. Parents become personally interested in helping their child understand how to cope more effectively with circumstances while staying cool, polite, and respectful of the child and themselves.

Allow Mistakes

Who were you told during your youth about the mistakes? Are these the messages, which you have? Poor errors. You should be making no mistakes. If you make errors, you are dumb, evil, incompetent, or a loser. Do not let people find out why you made an error. If they do, then give an argument even though it is not real. We name these "wild conceptions of mistake" because not only do they harm self-esteem, they often encourage frustration and discouragement. When you feel discouraged, it is hard to learn and grow. We all know people who made an error and then caved in to a hole trying to cover it up. They do not realize that people always really understand when they sincerely accept their faults, apologize, and attempt to fix the issues they made. (If lawmakers grasped this principle, wouldn't that be wonderful?)

Hiding errors leaves you alone, so you cannot correct secret mistakes or benefit from them. Trying to avoid errors leaves you tense and nervous. We have heard a saying: "Better judgment comes from practice, and knowledge comes from bad judgment" You have the ability to help your kids change these crazy mistaken notions. Say to your kids that every person in the world will carry on making mistakes for as long as they live. If this is so, it is more beneficial to see mistakes as chances to know, rather than declarations of inadequacy.

Teach the children to see mistake creation as a way to receive useful support from others. They will be ready to accept responsibility for what they have done, even though it has been a mistake because they know it does not mean they are bad or they are going to get into trouble. It means they are willing to be accountable, which is a necessary step to use mistakes as a learning opportunity. Sometimes errors require you to make corrections where possible, and at least to apologize when it is not possible to make amends. Inform your kids that error making is not as important as what they are doing about them. Anyone can make mistakes but it takes a secure person to say, "I'm wrong and I'm sorry." If a child wants to make corrections for a mistake, Mistakes' Three Rs of Recovery can help them do that.

1. Recognize the fault, with a feeling of obligation rather than guilt.

2. Reconcile when rendering an excuse to the ones you have disappointed or harmed.

3. Resolve the problem, by working together for a plan when possible.

The Three Rs of Recovery can help you make amends with your child if you make a mistake. In addition, note when you make errors do not hesitate to let them out. Your kids are going to really understand, and benefit from your modeling.

Methods to Foster Cooperation

Instructions are clear and simple. Kids cannot remember detailed tasks that include a couple of things to remember. 'Go and grab your shoes, coat, and gloves' includes three things you should remember. If he realizes one you will be lucky. So keep your inquiries easy and simple. If you want your child to help put away toys, understanding a specific request like 'let's put all your cars in the box' is much easier for him than a general instruction to 'clear up' when he does not know where to put things. Simple good outcomes. 'Let us put on your pajamas and then I'll read a story for you' gives the child a very clear indication of the sequence of events. The result must be something the child wants to do because it is used as a reward. If you listen carefully, you may find that you are actually saying, 'If you don't put on your pajamas, I won't read you a story,' which is a threat rather than a positive result. The trouble with this response to hazard is that there are two derogatory comments in it. It points out what the child should not do, and then threatens the withdrawal of a reward he has not yet had.

Negative motivation makes it difficult to cooperate happily. To state, the positive gives you a much more cooperative and warm interaction. Cooperation with control. That means keeping an eye on whether or not he does what you asked. We all make a request too often and then walk away because we have other things to do. Then, 10 minutes later, we find that the child has not done what we wanted and that we feel crossed that we were ignored. We have to stay throughout the whole process when teaching young children to cooperate, prompt them, and help them to do what we ask. Strengthen both efforts at teamwork. Young children are still not enough qualified to do just what we expect. They lose their attention, they forget what to do and they are quickly diverted from the mission. They need to be commended and congratulated for every effort they make to keep them motivated and keep them on the job. Prompts both physical and mental. They may need to be gently reminded or physically shown what to do to teach them and help them to cooperate. The task might have to be broken down into various components: 'Let's see if you can pick up the truck? 'And then, after he's finished something, 'Okay, that's fine, bring something in the package now.' Taking steps, supporting the child, and motivating the child to support you are both opportunities to improve it. Humor, rebellion, and rivalry. Humor and saying the opposite sometimes gets the desired effect. 'I don't really want you to put on your pajamas' may have a dramatic effect on a kid running about at bedtime without some clothing on. 'I bet you can't get into the car before Lucy' suddenly motivates a 3-year-old reticent, who does not want to go shopping. Similarly, counting to three will help a child concentrate on speeding or finishing the task.

Chapter 4: Avoiding Common Parenting Mistakes

Just like today's environment is unique, so are our children and youth. They are no longer reacting to parenting focused on terror. The old, fear-based strategies in turn undermine the power of a parent. The punishment threat only turns the children to stand against their parents and makes, the rebel. The coercion of yelling and physically abusing does not anymore create control but merely adorns the willingness of a child to listen and cooperate. Families are searching for improved contact with their children to brace them for today has heightened life stresses but, sadly, they are also utilizing obsolete approaches to parenting.

When parents yell at kids, it only dulls their hearing ability. The children of today require better communication skills to succeed at school and, more pertinently, to remain competitive in the free market or to grow professionally in a lasting relationship as they grow older. When children pay attention to their parents and parents pay attention to their children, these skills are most efficiently learnt. When parents learn how to respond to their children, children listen to their parents. What happens when you are listening to loud music? You lose hearing. The same happens all the time when parents are yelling or making demands. This has a distinct impact as parents nowadays scream or talk the way their parents did. Children are just going to be turned off today and parents are going to lose control.

Give Up Punishment

Societies have been marginalized, dominated, and abused by wealthy, punishing rulers in previous generations but today it is not so. Citizens are not likely to vote for racism and civil rights violations; rather, they should protest. People have given their freedom for political values. Children today will not be welcoming the possibility of retribution in a comparable manner. They are going to strike. Children now sense the cruelty of retribution more profoundly. This falls out as intensified opposition, anger, denial, and defiance as retribution goes in. Today, children ignore the principles of their parents, and at younger and younger age's revolt against parental authority. Until they are mentally stable or willing to let go of encouragement from their parents, children, and teens step apart and deny the help that is so vital to their growth. They hope to be safe from the influence of their parents at a period when they need the power to thrive healthily.

Children and teenagers refuse appropriate adult assistance until they are socially trained. Most parents understand that the old disciplinary techniques do not fit, they also do not know anyway. They are holding back from punishing, but that is not working either. Permitted parenting does not give parental control that the children need. Some kids take a mile when granted an inch of strength. Children learn to make easy use of their right to exploit and influence adults. They are in charge when children are permitted to make use of heavy, aggressive moods, emotions, and tantrums to get their way. When a child is in control, they are out of control of their parents. Across other cases, they can experience some of the same issues as children who are born with obsolete fear-based abilities. When kids are in control, they are out of control of their parents. Whether a child grows up with fear-based abilities or permissive abilities, if the child does not experience control of his parents, he will fight back or reject any attempts that parents can make to gain back or maintain control. Its development will be limited, disconnected from the support of his parents. By utilizing the Toddler Discipline techniques, parents will be able to offer their children the independence and guidance they need to build a good and balanced sense of self.

Consequences of Fear Centered Parenting

The traditional fear-based ways of handling our children by coercion, ridicule, rejection, and discipline not only have lost their control but also are ineffective. Children are more vulnerable than those of earlier generations are. They are eager to achieve far better but are often heavily affected by traditional discipline practices such as shouting, spanking, beating, bullying, detention, disapproving, insulting, and bullying. These strategies were useful when children were more dense-skinned but they are obsolete and detrimental today. Punishing kids by spanking has in the past made them fear power and obey the regulations. This has the reverse reaction today. Violence means outright violence. This is a more sensible symptom. Today's children can be more imaginative and wiser than in past generations, but they are often more affected by outer circumstances. As kids are more responsive, aggression implies overt abuse.

Today's children will know better to value others, not through methods of intimidation but through emulation. Children are trained to imitate their kin. Their minds often take photos, make videos to copy, and mimic anything you say or do. Practically they know this through emulation and teamwork.

Kids slowly understand how to treat people as adult's model polite behaviors. When parents learn to stay cool, calm, and affectionate while having to deal with a toddler throwing a tantrum, that child gradually understands to stay cool, calm, and loving when strong feelings come up. Parents should stay calm, quiet, caring, and compassionate while studying what to do when kids get out of reach.

When children get out of balance, parents should remain calm and relaxed while knowing what to do. When you beat kids to gain back advantage, kids realize that when they get out of reach, violence is the solution. I have seen a mother hit her son many times, saying, "Stop attacking your brother." She wants him to know how it feels, but attacking is not the answer. She bolsters his proclivity to hit or use violence by hitting her son. Later he would inevitably return to acting out his frustration through either overt or passive violence if he does not get what he needs. Though spanking or whacking kids worked for decades, today it has backfired. Fear-based parenting strategies hinder the normal growth of our children and make our task less rewarding and more time-consuming as parents.

4.1 Coping with Toddler Problems

Food wars are a fact of living for young people. Around a fifth of moms believe their preschooler has an eating disorder. They may be fussy over what their kid consumes, or whether he does not eat enough, but that is always raising worry. Particularly mothers feel very affectionately concerned with how and what their child eats. This relates to the early months of breastfeeding- and bottle-feeding where she was mostly responsible for feeding the baby. Checking the amount the baby feeds and related to how the baby grows and thrives is very much the role of the mother and it is too easy for her to feel blamed if her baby does not grow well enough.

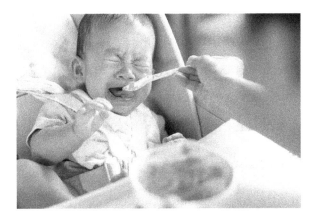

Weaning

Taking your baby through weaning is just another hurdle the

first year overcomes. Some babies will accept, some will not. In addition, the alacrity spoon while others resist, spit, struggle and cause trouble and distress. Babies generally begin to be weaned sometime between the ages of 4 and 6 months. There is no need to do so. As your baby becomes used to the new idea and new sensations it can be done gradually. A tiny taste of puree is often the starting point on your finger before a feed. Even blending some breast milk with baby rice is an early first step that allows your baby to use a familiar taste to manage a new texture. Stepping up the amount given and switching to a spoon while the kid is comfortable makes the transition easy. Babies have a very strong tongue thrust when they are primarily feeding teat since it's those tongue reflexes that help strip the milking teat. So do not worry if everything you seem to get into your baby's mouth with the tongue thrust keeps coming out again. That does not mean that your kid does not like the meal; it is just that he has not known how to hold the meal in his mouth.

Quitting Breastfeeding

When you decide to go back to work within the first six months of your infant, you'll need to show him how to move it to a bottle; if it's beyond that period, you'll just be willing to pass it straight to a teacher beaker and skip it. Even at this young age, change can be resisted, but if you keep the faith, he will cope. Perhaps the main concern is the feeling of remorse or frustration over trying to make a transition until you know he is able to do so. You may also feel sad that the special phase is ending. Some mothers do not have to make this decision and carry on breastfeeding into their second and third years. They are able to wait before their kid says he will not breast-feed any more. Whatever itinerary you choose, you need to feel at ease. I have seen mothers who are eager to avoid breastfeeding their babies but feel the demands of the child are too intense. Most mothers were able to maintain breastfeeding, but without a healthy diet, their child will not grow enough, so constant breast-on-demand snacking limits the infant's hunger for some other food. It is important to strike a balance, so you and the needs of your child are met. You should take care of this case because you are liable for breast and food exposure. Your child requires a healthy diet to satisfy his or her nutritional needs. He would not be willing to do anything as an infant and as a toddler: you have to do that for him.

Shifting To Healthy Foods

Proceeding towards the end of the first year to try different food textures is another transition that can create issues. Some babies stop going earlier on to lumpy pure 'e. We vomit out lumps, cough, and decline to consume anything except the creamy pure 'e with which we have been accustomed. They need to know how to work comfortably and without gagging with soft lumps of food. Reducing the pure liquid content makes it stickier. Mashing soft root vegetables will render the pure 'e more textured so the kid will not notice a pea or a bit of carrot in the center of the pure 'e' which is also an issue for stage 2 container foods. The more subtle shift of texture also works and helps your child respond to the different food demands of his mouth.

At the end of the first year, finger foods are typically implemented at providing little bits of biscuit, rusk, or cooked soft potato that your child can pick up and consume with his mouth. Much of this should vanish in a game built to involve you in picking it up off the bottom of the tray on the board. If you whisk it off to the bin because it is dirty, you will find howls of consternation until he finds the next bit to start throwing to the ground. This is a chance for your baby to explore the texture and feel it. He wants to crush the rice, create a mess, enjoy himself completely and clean his fingers afterward. Through this process, he will begin to put food in his mouth. The first solid foods should be those that dissolve in saliva to a paste. Rusks and rich tea biscuits are ideal since the baby has the idea of sucking something strong but there are no pieces that can make him gag. He may bite off pieces as he becomes more adventurous, but they will quickly dissolve in his mouth. If you consume your meal with him, you will be able to offer tastes from your plate and thus broaden his taste and texture experience without especially cooking for him.

Self-indulgence

If you want to, you can truly interrupt and interfere with self-feeding development. If you are trying to stop the mess, keep cleaning your baby's hands, and face as he is feeding, he will eventually realize that making dirty hands is not a smart thing before become nervous about handling food itself. Then he might be unwilling to pick up food in his hands but does not have enough experience to handle cutlery well. He will then resorts to being spoon-fed by you, and there tends to be a more passive and childish trend. So seek to wait until you wash your child's face and hands until the end of the meal. It is supposed to be a signal that the meal is over, no mess. The other way to interrupt this self-feeding transition is to fight over the spoon. Parents who are worried about the amount their child eats like to stay in charge of the spoon because then they understand how much their child eats instead of tipping into his bib or smearing on the tray. However, your toddler will want to take charge of himself towards the end of the first year. During any mealtime, there is always an odd cycle with many spoons: you have one or two, and he has one or two; others get tossed into the floor; but typically much of the food ends up in his mouth, either on your spoon or on his. Stacking his spoon for him can help, and gently guiding his hand to make sure it gets into his mouth with food still on, if he will let you, it is an art. When you continue arguing for spoon power, you can realize you have a kid that fails to comply and does not feed because he is angry and irritated

Temper Tantrums

Temper tantrums are representative of infants, though some kids hold them on for several years if they find that they are a way to get whatever they want. Most often, children throw a hissy fit when they are very stressed, starving irritably, physically exhausted, or sound ill. As your child becomes more "knowing," outbursts may just be her way of pushing the boundaries of seeing how you are going to respond. Kids still choose to cry and whine at the worst possible moments. You may drive your car, go grocery shopping, eat at a steakhouse or a friend's place and she does just when you would least suspect your child to make a scene. We incline to want to get her to stop doing something right away. We are ashamed and our degree of tension is high. That is because parents often turn to intimidation and prohibitions. Rather, we need to recognize that the tantrum signifies something, so the only way that helps is to get to the underside of it and attempt to meet the needs of the child.

Types of Tantrums

There is a major difference between temper tantrums and one hurled by a kid who is angry, frustrated, and who tests the limits. The very first type of tantrum necessitates little more than a parent who determines the cause, remains calm and upbeat, and helps with food, rest, or comfort. While it may be awkward to have a child weeping incoherently in a supermarket or on a social occasion, there is at least a physiological situation underpinning the hissy fit, which can be quickly resolved once you discover it out. In addition, when you do your best to be in control you will ultimately be.

The second category of tantrum is like any conflict overpower. It is less than an articulation of your child's way of trying to proclaim some authority in a circumstance in which she feels powerless. Know when kids say "No! "In addition, they are attempting to convey something to you, or throw a temper tantrum. You have to be cool, stand back, and try to find out what the secret meaning it could be that all you need to listen to. Children occasionally feel frustrated just like grown-ups, because they feel nobody is paying attention to them.

Resolving Them

Often it may be tough to say for sure what a temper tantrum is mostly about because small children are unable to describe the question. Most parents, however, learn to identify symptoms and may make a prediction. If you believe that the behavior of your child is the product of being starving, get some nutrition for her to consume as quickly as practical, even though it is not her normal mealtime. It is a good idea to bring with you some kind of quick lunch just for such emergencies. If you think your child is excessively tired, reduce your conversation and talk in a smooth voice, keep or rock her, as well as end up taking her to her bedroom or anywhere she can relax as soon as possible. If you know your kid is ill, speak with a sweet voice, reassuring her quietly. See if someone near the area can get you an empty crockery or trash can, and a warm washcloth, if you think she will vomit. Do arrangements as patiently as possible if she needs medical help. If you have been otherwise involved, talk with a friend at the breakfast table or on the phone for a long time; make sure you pay a lot of attention to your toddler when you are done. Some kids struggle with transformations, and this can give rise to a tantrum in itself. If you are at the play area, for example, let your kid know ahead of time that you are going to leave soon. "We are going to have to go back in 15 minutes. Would you like to go down some more of the slide, or swing? "The reminder and the choice in advance will allow your baby better manage moves. If your kid tests the limits clearly, stay calm, and resist getting into a fight. Speak in a soothing voice; let her know gently that whilst you understand she gets mad, this is still the law. For starters, "I know you want to still linger at the playground here, but we've got to get home to have lunch."

Avoiding drawbacks

Family life often has patterns. Recognize if you can pinpoint any frequent tantrum triggers then try avoiding them. For example, if when you go shopping your child appears to get tantrums, leave her with your spouse, or a sitter. Children often act when plans abruptly change, and if this is the situation with your child, plan ahead of time and stick to it. Illustrate the boundaries already when you do anything to your kid. For instance, if you go to the supermarket and your child wants to purchase a toy, inform her in advance what you are going to agree to and adhere to it. Do not give in to the attempts made by children to get you back down, if they are complaining, demanding, or trying to trick the situation. It may work to distract an infant with a match at the first indication of a tantrum. If she does not calm down, however, detach by sitting down to read or move outside the entrance, letting her know you're waiting to give a cuddle as soon as she's ready for it. Even people are attempting to overdo it. Young children prefer habits and get upset and weary when they were sweeping from one exercise to another. It is unavoidable occasionally, so consider hard and long before you sign up for baby yoga, dance classes, or some other prearranged courses. Racing from one action to the next raises stress levels for everyone and sets the stage for emotional outbursts.

Tips for Coping

There are many things you should remember when you have a tantrum at your child:

• Do not turn to violence by hitting your child or spanking her. That is the surest means of training her to be abusive against others.

• Do not attempt to physically restrain a child unless it is about to run out of traffic or harm itself in some other very direct and tangible manner.

• Should not respond to intimidation or prohibitions. These simply do not work when children are also being unreasonable, and they only spiral out of control the already started emotional turmoil.

• Argue not. You cannot win a debate with an irrational person. • Do not try to make your child embarrassed or ridicule her behavior. In the future, this teaches her to cuss out at others.

• Don't attempt to handle the temper tantrum in general. Take your child to a place where you can be isolated, and speak privately. This is polite to others and makes the situation easier for you to handle.

Dealing with an Aggressive Child

There is a difference between experiencing a feeling and displaying emotions, such as a temper tantrum. Anger is a feeling that follows the belief that you cannot get what you want, or that you are powerless in a situation. It can also be a cover-up for hurt feelings. Children who seem angry may be frustrated with their parents, other children, themselves, life, or other people who are angry with them. Children may think that no one is paying attention to them or considering their needs. Children usually have good reasons for feeling angry, even if they do not know what those reasons are. When children are bossed and controlled and have no choices, they will probably feel angry. Children who are overprotected often feel angry. If adults abuse children either physically or verbally, children will feel angry. In addition, if a child sees his parent reacting to a display of angry feelings by being aggressive, he will do the same. Parents often respond to anger and aggression with more attempts to control and with intimidation, making the situation worse. If you or your child feels angry, there may be a power struggle going on, and it is important to disengage from the power contest and work for cooperation.

Cause of Aggressive or Unruly Behavior

There are obvious explanations why today's children become more unruly, arrogant, hostile, and abusive in both their homes and classrooms. This is not a huge mystery. This causes hyperactivity in boys — or what is often known as Attention Deficit Disorder — when they are over-stimulated by violence or the prospect of discipline at home. In girls, aggressive tendencies with feelings of low self-esteem and disordered eating are acted out against themselves. Go into any prison and you will find that all violent offenders have been punished severely or beaten as children, without exception. The brutality they have endured is devastating almost as tragic is the cruelty they have committed upon their families. However, just beyond the jails and at the counseling center, as a consequence of fear-based upbringing, many millions of people suffer from stress, anxiety, apathy, and other mental illnesses. On the other hand, today many children are disruptive and impeded by the "soft" parenting affections. Conservative parents are right to be cautious of new approaches to soft parenting. Even though the purpose to be love-based is apparent, there is no practice of the skills to make it successful. The independence and influence provided by the five signals must be matched by similarly strong abilities to retain an advantage over children and build harmony. When you want to drive a good vehicle, you will make sure you have excellent braking. You cannot offer any independence to children when you have the expertise to control them and act in an organized way.

You cannot offer any independence to children when you

have the expertise to control them and act in an organized way. Many parents who had been mistreated as children never decided to beat, spank, abuse, or threaten their offspring. They knew what wasn't working, and stopped doing it, to be responsible humans. The problem is they did not know how to substitute love-based skills for the old fear-based practices. For several instances, failing to punish their parents has ruined their family. This kind of soft discipline is just as unsuccessful as conventional methods focused on anxiety. Giving up past tactics built on fear just works when you substitute them with something new, which is more successful. Though kids today have different needs, they do need a managed adult. Otherwise, the kid goes out of reach no matter how much you love your kids. Positive discipline includes the idea of making the infant take time out to eliminate the urge to spank or threaten in a number of situations that are suitable with maturity. Then, the final step is time outs. There are plenty of other techniques to be incorporated even before having to resort to time out, ensuring that time out succeeds. Otherwise, it becomes just another fear-based punishment and loses its efficacy

Suggestions

Validate your child's feelings, "You're angry. It's okay to feel angry, but can you tell me in words instead of actions who or what you are angry about?" Wait for the child's response and listen with interest instead of saying, "You shouldn't be angry." Sometimes children cannot identify their feelings when they are upset. Let your child know it is okay to wait a while and to talk with you as soon as he is ready. You can help your child defuse her anger by finding out (perhaps through guessing) what she wants and helping her obtain it, such as, "You're angry because your sister gets to stay up later and you wish you could, too. When you are her age, you'll be able to stay up as late as she does." Do not choose sides when your children fight because this is one of the primary triggers for children's anger. Instead, put them in the same boat and say, "Kids, I see you are having a hard time working this out. You can take some time to cool off and try again later, or you can both finish this fight somewhere else, or you can work it out here, but I'm not taking sides." If you have children who argue, try letting them have the last word or hugging them instead of arguing back. Ask your children for their opinions instead of telling them what to do. When you recognize a power struggle, stop and say, "I don't want to control you, but I would appreciate your help. Let's see what we can work out after we calm down." If your child is hurting others with his aggressive behavior, let him know you realize he may be feeling hurt and upset about something, but you cannot let him hurt others. If your child is young enough, remove him from the situation and sit with him, helping him talk about what he is upset about. If he is older, say, "I love you. Come get me when you are ready to talk and then leave. If children need to sit down together to work out a problem, sit with them while they talk.

Avoid reacting to aggression with aggression, which creates a power struggle and models the opposite of what you hope to achieve. Also, avoid reinforcing aggression by giving in to it. Look for areas where frustration can be tempting. Would you put your nose into the life of your baby, including lecturing on schoolwork, peers, shoes, etc.? Do you nag your family, rather than setting up routines and using tracking? Will you use retribution rather than seeking solutions? Will you render recommendations, rather than demands? Children react to "It's time to have dinner" better than "Come to the table now." Establish family gatherings so your kids realize there are a spot and time every week that they can chat about stuff that concerns them, are listened to, and discuss answers to problems that benefit everyone.

Give up on Rhetorical Questions

Far more than using the hypothetical phrases "should you" and "should you?" When you try to make a point in a persuasive speech, rhetorical questions are fine, but they are counterproductive when you ask for the cooperation. There is always an implied message to every rhetorical question. The implied message in parenting is usually a negative message of guilt, which a loving parent would not want to say directly. It is inferred, then, in a verbal letter. Many mothers do not even realize that they are giving a negative message but it is easy to recognize with a little soul-searching. Women will use rhetorical questions particularly to motivate children to be submissive. When a mum wants her child to clean up his room instead of saying, "Would you clean up your room, please? "By first using a rhetorical statement she throws in a little shame and guilt like," Why is this room still a mess? "What it could imply is," You should have cleaned this space. You are bad. You are a dirt bag. You do not listen to me the way you should, etc. Mothers increase their chance of creating cooperation by having to give up rhetorical questions before sending a suggestion; otherwise, children just stop listening. Not only does avoiding rhetorical questions help to create cooperation, but it also prevents your kids from becoming exposed to poor communication skills. Not only do hypothetical questions not work for the infant but they also discourage parents from simply accepting blame for the harmful messages they send out. It is hard to understand why our children are not willing to cooperate with us without clearly recognizing our hateful thoughts.

Being straightforward, particularly with little boys, is one of the most valuable skills mothers need to acquire. Women will often state what they are disappointed about, but with a request, they do not follow. This is like desert fishing. We have no hope of getting the response we want. Here are some examples of how not to be direct:

- You kids make so big of a racket. -- Be calm

- Your space is just another disaster-Tidy up your place.

Being Direct

The parent attempts to encourage the kid to do something by focusing on the issue in each of these examples but is not asking him to do anything. Perhaps the implicit question is not even understood by the boy, who is doing nothing but staring into space. The message must be straightforward without focussing on the derogatory term to get a clear answer. Focusing on what a child has done wrong or whether a child would feel guilty does not help to create cooperation. Let us discuss ways to rephrase offensive feedback as powerful calls for practice. Rather than suggesting the kids create too much noise, suggest you would be silent, please? Instead of suggesting that your space is yet another disaster, should you suggest to clean your room up?

Easy Ways to End Baby Whining and Parental Bargaining

Have you ever happened to meet someone that is more stubborn than a child attempting to get what she desires is? Well, there is no one more driven or committed than a kid on a quest to get acceptance from his or her parent.

Unfortunately, this degree of determination is not always adequately embraced by mothers who are frequently pushed into these inappropriate moments of hostage talks – in the grocery store's chocolate row, in Walmart's toy aisle, while trying to prepare dinner or attempting to take a bath. It is almost as if kids can see when we are vulnerable and are trying to pounce in our weaker moments. While teaching children gratitude is important in combating the desperate pleas in the stores, it is equally crucial to eliminate the negotiations when they are out of control. From common questions like, "Are we still here? "Can I have cake for breakfast this weekend? "Can I have candy for a snack this afternoon? "Children are renowned for their one-track brains, so they are going to ask ... and ask ... and just continuously ask ... only if you have reversed your plans at the last minute. Why do kids display nagging behavior? As mentioned in the previous parts of this book, for every behavior, to resolve it properly, you should first acknowledge the root of the problem.

Baby nagging is a learned trait that children of any age may engage in. Children will continue to do it because when, in a moment of stupidity, you relented and let them stay up for an extra couple minutes after the ninth time, they insisted. In brief, the pestering worked- achieving the child's goal of prolonged bedtime. This tends to happen because feelings of hopelessness or loneliness stashed away from earlier encounters crop up and take over in the possibility of the end of the good times. The emotions may come from earlier today or from as far away as infancy — they linger in the mind of the child and are put into question through simple moments of everyday life.

Whining Kids Don't Try To Exploit You

When your kid whines, he is not out to get you. Just he does not want you to give up on unreasonable demands. He is trying to show he has your support.

He has decided to want something unreasonable, so you will say a soft, firm "No." Then he will be able to open up bad feelings. He will eventually shed the emotions when he is weeping. Ultimately, if you listen, he will appreciate your presence, appreciate your affection, and feel a lot better of himself and his life. He will cease to need what he was weeping for since he has you. Seek to capture him saying, "I want a cookie," but actually meaning, "Just say 'no.' I need a strong hug with your arms surrounding me!"

Give Closeness and Clear Limit If He Is Not Satisfied

The cold tone used by most of us when we say, "No," helps to make a kid feel even more lost and floating in an indifferent universe. It intensifies the rut in which your child whines.

If you can say, "Nope, no cookies anymore! Tomorrow might be! "Your child receives touch from you with a wide smile and a peck on the cheek instead of cookies. When he whines a little bit more, you could come back and say, "Nah, nah, nah, nah!" In addition, stroke his face, ending with just a little kiss. When he continues, offer him even more love, "I am your cookie with chocolate chip! I am all for you! "A big smile. So round him throw your arms and pick him up. To some point, the love that you give will tip him either to laugh or to a tantrum.

Dealing with Toddler Hyperactivity

Among many parents, there is a lot of anxiety that their infants may have ADHD. This term, 'attention deficit hyperactivity disorder,' has become a common diagnosis among older children of school age and replaces the term 'hyperactive' because it is more accurate in its description. ADHD is a psychological disorder of a particular childhood behavioral disorder and every diagnostic category must exclude and include cases. The question to parents is the exclusion point. You may have a kid who has attention problems and is very overactive but may not fulfill the specific diagnostic requirements. That does not erase the reality that you are living with a kid who is complicated to treat and tires you out. This category of diagnosis does not apply to preschool children, either. Young children display such a broad variety of rates of behavior and attention that specifically diagnosing this condition in this age category has been challenging. Another feature of a mental health label such as ADHD is that it links to a specific treatment found to be valuable. The drugs were found to be particularly good

Beneficial for older children with ADHD but not generally prescribed below the age of six. So we are faced with a scenario where we need to look closely at the behavior of young children in a variety of contexts, and about their stage of development. With this age group of preschoolers, we do not pursue a diagnostic category. However, it is obvious that ADHD does not erupt suddenly at age 6: the signs will be there earlier in childhood.

Paying Heed and Concentration

Attention and concentration are essential skills that enable a child to learn. It is very hard to learn anything new if you end up losing your concentration every few minutes or if you cannot attend the task long enough to get to the end. Yet, as you may know, in the pre-school years, children's focus and commitment are minimal, so it is by a combination of teaching so maturation that children will expand these forces when they get older. Your 1-year-old would be flitting around the toy bin, tossing it over, picking up a few items for a couple of minutes, mouthing them, and then exchanging them for something special. However, if he really is interested and can end up making up a game to go with it, your 3-year-old would be able to sit and play with a teddy bear for up to half an hour. The concern is that there are no specific rules as to how long children will be able to concentrate on growing level. Psychological assessments of the rates of development in adolescents are far more linked to what they can accomplish compared to how they do so. The thing is, the focus is always associated with curiosity and inspiration. Your 2-year-old will be able to hold still and listen to a story when it's told with amusing sounds, in a book with plenty of illustrations to make him entertained and less lonely at the end of the day sitting on your lap. However, if he is distracted, and you are trying to make him sit still to listen to a dull tale that does not have any images, I wonder how long he would last. So many specific problems influence the attention of young children that making some clear guidance is quite challenging.

While becoming straightforward on what you expect him to be willing to achieve, you will help improve the child's capacity to learn and persevere through tasks. If his flitting stops him from carrying out certain tasks, then think about the above list and schedule those basic things you realize he loves. Check how long he will keep on track and then, if he drops ahead, quickly places it to one foot. After playing with some other toys, encourage him to come back and join the task once more. He can slowly understand that he can complete a job like a puzzle and achieve a sense of achievement and contentment. You can seek to May his desire to keep performing the job for a minute or two longer because you know how long he will continue. You will slowly build up the duration of his focus period. One of the biggest reasons parents complain over their child's attention span is because they do not want to listen to what is being discussed while he is bad. You order him to go to get his hat, but he runs off and then does something else; he will not sit down for meals at the table; he runs off at bedtime and will not be returned to bed. Sometimes it is very hard to know if your child is just disobedient, or if he has not heard the instruction. It is necessary to make sure your kid listened and recognized what you asked. Young children have limited memory for a list of steps. A 2-year-old can obey a clear command like 'place the cup on the table,' and a 4-year-old can obey a directive to perform three items in sequence with one directive like 'place this cup on the table, put the spoon with the drawer and get me a plate' – that's why they feel cooperative. We often embed one instruction inside another as parents, which can confuse young children. We need to learn to be clear and concise in our demands, using language that our kids can understand and not adding in additional information that just makes them forget what we asked. To make sure you get his attention and compliance, make sure he looks at you when you ask him to do something, remove his distractions for him, encourage him to repeat what you've said, and see if he does what you're asking.

4.2 Techniques of French Parenting

You do not need an interpreter when it comes to parenting in France to tell you there are significant differences between how Americans and Europeans raise their children. Children from France could seem to be just born with je ne sais quoi, but as the author and ex-pat from France, Florence Mars says, it is because they have been raised to be extremely well behaved. (Oh, excellently dressed exquisitely, too.)

1. The Pause of Two Minutes

Pamela Druckerman, an American writer residing in Paris, reported in her book "Bringing up Bebe" that most babies in France sleep longer as early as two months old. Although some may consider this finding, questionable, pediatric experts relate this trend to a French parenting pattern, which is often referred to as the "two-minute delay."

In this process, when babies startle awake screaming or make a sound at night, the mothers give the baby about two minutes to see if the baby can resolve anything that has disturbed him or her. Only if, in those few minutes, the baby seems unable to soothe himself back to sleep, the parents will then attend him. While this may seem somewhat unorthodox and runs counter to normal mothering instincts, pediatric experts explain that newborns have two-hour cycles of sleep and the two- pause educates them to link these phases of sleep. If a mother or father sees the baby instantly when the baby cries between these phases at night, it will be more difficult for the baby to learn how and when to connect the cycles. What could make things much worse is that the child is now becoming dependent on an older person to relieve him or her back to bed.

2. Dining Manners

One of the most widely respected behaviors of French children is that they appear to have no trouble consuming 'adult 'food. While a fair number of non-French parents usually believe that children prefer hotdogs, sandwiches, chicken nuggets or fries to regular meal fares, French babies, on the other hand, at a very young age, are exposed to a variety of foods. There is no such thing as kiddie food or adult food to French parents but just fruit. Druckerman reflected on how she learned how special her child was to French kids when dining at a restaurant, in one part of her novel. She noted how behaved the other kids were enjoying their food on their high chairs, while her kid was giving her all kinds of problems, and be all picky and attempting to make so much fuss. The writer also learned that French household mealtimes for the family were also strictly observed. She surmised the early access in French children to several foods and close observance of meal times ingrain table discipline. This results in them being second nature to good table manners.

3. Teaching Patience

This aspect of French parenting is somehow associated with the two previous topics, which have already been mentioned. One commonly lauded behavior of French children is that they are rarely seen throwing tantrums in public. Besides disciplining children, French mothers also teach the virtue of patience to their children. Children would also try opportunities to get their parents to cede to their demands. One way to get parents to say " yes "is by wearing them away with prolonged nagging and grumbling.

Child psychologists suggest adults that they should not be

punishing children for their poor behavior. Not only does it encourage them to do it again but it also provides them a modicum of authority. When French parents say no "or" wait to their children, they both assume and mean it. Unlike many other parenting methods that give way to bargaining with your offspring, much of the time the French will not even consider the notion. Which teaches French children to be careful at a young age. This type of patience training is thought to sometimes help children become more composed as they get older.

4. Spanking or La Fessee

Particularly other families from neighboring nations sometimes perceive French parents as being too strict and authoritarian with their children, this might be valid to some degree because French parents often favor la Fessee, or spanking, to the more common discipline methods that promote "simple behavioral moulding." That is, of course, also a sophisticated way of suggesting that parents will make their children a little slacker. Nevertheless, French parents should educate their students on the concept of power as early as possible, and encourage them to comply with their laws. They do not utilize la Fessee right off the bat, as authoritative and inflexible as French parents might seem. A strong 'No! 'Or stop, serve as a warning for children to be misbehaved, followed by 'it's enough!' or 'it's enough! 'For successful practice. The spanking component is expected during the child's earlier part of development and training. However, as the children learn these steps, the "ça suffit!" aspect will often suffice to get them to act.

5. Balance

Parents everywhere are obsessed with keeping a harmony between home and working life — for the French this juggling act is viewed as essential to the welfare of the entire family. It is seen as equally problematic to cater to children at the cost of family or work, or to overemphasize a job over family. This ideology goes into effect during pregnancy, when "France's point isn't that anything goes. It's that young ladies should be relaxed and reasonable." Children and their gadgets do not overtake a French home, and motherhood is not seen as the central identity of a woman; it is just one important element.

6. Disagreeing viewpoints

As can be anticipated, there will always be those who do not agree with the French parenting style. One British lifestyle writer said French parents should not believe their children to be their peers, but they are only little human beings who are all ready to be designed and shaped by the state school system. This trend of conduct exhibited by French children is mainly attributed to their school environment under which they are kept for as long as 10-12 hours in a state-run local crèche, where they have little alternative but to become confident and sociable.

It will be naïve of course to think that the French parenting style will extend in any context or location. Our societies, feeling of togetherness, religion, and social norms were always the greatest influential variables in the diverse parenting styles. What works for parents in France will not always work for others, and vice versa. However, parents are guided by a religious obligation to fulfill their duties in the best possible way. Evaluating what works with many communities, such as the French with an example, is one-way parents can become the best they can be with their babies. Hence, it is recommended that you decide what works best for your child.

American vs French Parenting

There are few items that have not entered the French lifestyle misconception — which says all the French do, from cooking to carrying clothing to putting on weddings. This applies to upbring, however, predictably. However, as it turned out, the methodology between parents in France however their American equivalents is very distinctive. Read on to test what they are.

French parents gave their children tight boundaries.

In the book "Bringing up Bebe," writer Pamela Druckerman explained that, from an early age, French parents have strong standards on what is anticipated and what is inappropriate behavior from their children. It provides an authoritarian form of leadership that leaves no doubt over who is in charge of the household.

French kids know the magic of four terms.

They say "hello" any time they walk into a room. Throughout the US, children usually know two "magic phrases," which are "thank you" and "please." According to "Bringing up Bebe," French kids learn four — "s'il vous plaît" (please), "merci" (thank you), "bonjour" (hello), and "au revoir" (goodbye). Although it is nice to tell welcome people in the US, it is important in France. In "Bringing up Bebe," Druckerman notes that, in France, "saying bonjour honors the dignity of the other individual." Therefore, it is necessary.

Children enjoy grown-up meals.

Throughout France, the idea of a "children's menu" or "kid's meal" — which appears to be cornerstone throughout American restaurants — is not as traditional. There is very little difference between what may be on a parent or child's tray, as per the book "French Kids Eat Anything."

Kids are given solid, refined tastes from an early age (think of Roquefort cheese and pate), which allows them room to cultivate a palate for foods that their American peers would consider "rude."

Children consume vegetables as well.

"French Kids Eat Everything" also shows how French parents want their children to consume vegetables. Obviously, when children are hungry, vegetables are typically served at the beginning of a meal, which means that they are more encouraged to eat them.

There is not as much variation in the hairstyles of French girls.

As per the book "Tell Bonjour to the Lady: Parenting from Paris to New York," French parents prefer to make their children stay with one look — a traditional bob — however, children can have any hairstyle in the United States.

Kids in France sleep all night.

Druckerman explains the French parents incorporate something called "The Pause" in "Bringing up Bebe." It is a strategy in which mothers pause a couple of minutes before reacting to their infant whenever they hear them continue to scream, which allows them an opportunity to "self-soothe." With time, this will teach children to sleep alone during the night.

The French children follow the timetables of their parents.

American parents frequently notice that their children's hobbies, such as baseball games, piano lessons, and tutoring sessions consume their weekends. As per "Say Bonjour to the Lady: Parenting from Paris to New York," French families base their weekends around themselves and merely carry their kids along, or have them do their own thing if they are old enough.

At a younger age, French children are granted further responsibilities.

In France, children are granted significantly more independence and accountability than children of their own ages in the US. As per the Huffington Post, it is normal for children in France to start walking down the road to school by age seven on their own and by age 11-ride public transport alone.

French children consume fewer treats compared with American girls.

According to "Growing up Bebe," French parents usually follow a regimen in which children consume three meals a day, including one afternoon snack.

American kids have more personality.

Megan Cradle wrote in The Atlantic that the stern, authoritarian form of parenting prevalent in France might often veer on the side of being too severe. It can mitigate hissy fits and meticulous eaters, which may leave no space to expose their creativity to French youngsters.

French parents are often at odds over the parental methods.

Guilt tends to be a typical by-product of American upbringing in many ways. (Possibly, because there is a thriving industry in the states devoted to showing that everything American family members do is unambiguously wrong.) In France, parents are less required to do anything and be anything, and parents are less inclined to feel bad for how they educate their babies, according to Today.

French parents never use feeding as bribery or bribe.

The French parents do not use food as a lure, threat, or incentive, according to "French Kids Consume Anything." This allows French children to establish positive relational connections with other forms of food which may prevent them from consuming it (or, in certain instances, may allow them to binge on it), which can contribute to a better overall diet and lifestyle.

French parents are not using as many books for parenting.

When you seek to use the aid of a book to parent like the French, you might have skipped the argument already. The parenting books are not as that in France as they are in the US, according to Today. Rather, parents using their intuition and other culturally approved strategies that have helped build a more unified parenting style throughout the country.

4.3 Practical Tips for a Better Relationship with Your Toddler

We would all like to be decent fathers and excellent mothers, but what does this mean? Providing a healthy house, decent food, good safety, a caring atmosphere, stimulating schooling, and socializing and playing benefits; But beyond that, we would like to know if we are making the right decisions and doing them? Is there really a correct way to raise kids? Are we doing our children's emotional and psychological harm by saying things that may come across to them as demeaning or punishing?

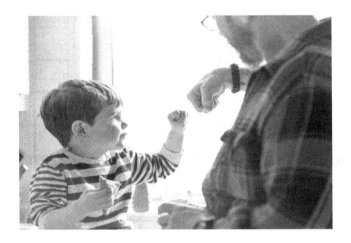

When we look back on the past 100 years on parental involvement advice, wonderful changes have occurred in the perceptions and trends of childcare and child nurturing. There are variations all over the world, across various cultural societies and classes. There is clearly no one perfect solution, but childcare patterns evolve in responding to the demands of the society into which the child is born. Currently, most kids in British society are conceived into a nuclear family system with limited interaction with the wider family and state dependence for health, education, and social support. The nature of family life has shifted significantly, as the rate of divorce has grown, and often babies are raised into complicated stepfamily systems and grow up in them. Too many adults and caregivers, how we handle divorce and reconstructed family life is a problem. We simply expect perfect babies, leading to an increment in the number of Caesarean section deliveries by up to 20 percent. We are also essential citizens in a culture that aims to uphold civil dignity, equity, and freedom of expression. Therefore, we need to think about what needs to grow up in such a social structure and be effective as parents. Think of how you interpret China's provision of getting just one child per household. How do you think the next generation would be influenced and how they act and socialize? You need to reflect on the values within each family that you believe is meaningful to you. Only then do you understand how you want to educate your babies, what behavior, what principles you want to instill, and carry on to coming generations. Are you aware of the values that you hold? Do you realize what helps you feel motivated? One thing, which seems clear to many parents, is that, although it takes so much time and effort, financial and vocational success may not be the only crucial feature of life. At the end of the day, satisfying marriages, stable family life, care for one another, and compassion is much more important and rewarding. And we ought to think how best to have our babies develop up with a sense of love for each other, to be willing to have meaningful and fulfilling connections with each other, to have true friends, and ultimately to develop long-lasting long term relationships such that the next century is safe and well cared for.

Fears and Discrepancies

Being a parent requires understanding how to deal with confusion. It is a struggle to transition to the next identity as it expands and evolves. Many parents find that their kid has already managed to move to the next stage, as they try to work with and evolve to one development stage. You just handle your day with two naps a day around your baby and then you suddenly find that he is on one nap a day and meal is not going to fit in because either he is too tired to eat or it is too early or too late. It at least keeps you on your feet and you can grow complacent at no time.

Parenthood is a path of guilt that never ends. You can even feel in someone's eyes that what you are doing is wrong. This is partially due to the juggling act many people undergo attempting to balance job or education with parenthood, various children's needs, children's needs against the husband, and children's and partner's needs toward self. Guilt is an emotion that is rather harmful, it may be crippling. Working or not working is always one of the most challenging decisions mothers make. We have a very potent ability to assert one's own choices by seeking parallel choices that match one's own and by ignoring the opposite. If you decide to go to work while your kid is a kindergartner for your own health, or you need to go to work for serious financial reasons, so you should recognize that reason to yourself and pick the greatest alternative care commitments that you can afford for your children. The most damaging method is to return to work, and then feel regretful about staying at home. It will kill you. It will demolish your connection with your kids, as you reward them for not being outside during the day. It will wreck your tasks. Moms who feel bad for having to work that hold their kids up at night and instead feel resentful and tired because they do not get enough sleep themselves to perform well throughout the day. Fathers arriving late from work could expect the kids to be kept up to see them and proceed to make them cheerful or over-excited before they are expected to sleep. If your interests have become more relevant than the interests of your infant, then that can contribute to confusion, distorted emotional responses, and more shame. Be explicit about your choices, and their causes. Lists of benefits and drawbacks will be useful but must be factual. There are also two aspects of a choice so do the best you can under certain situations and now. If you find it does not work or is incorrect for you and your family, you can always alter it later. However, make no decision and then continue to regret it and do nothing about it.

Understanding Your Child's Personality

An important aspect is understanding your child's personality if you are trying to improve your relationship with him or her. So, were you the kid who ran into class when you were young, excited to be there, or were you hesitant? Were you the much famous, or sometimes alone, in class? Have you enjoyed team sports from a very young age, or preferred reading a book? Perhaps one of the most daunting aspects we understand, as parents are that our children are not ourselves. You may be amazed at the notable differences between your character and that of your child, or perhaps the behavior of your child reminds you of something you wish you could change in your own personality. Every single one of us is distinctive: parent, child, and grandparent. We have various preferences, temperaments, and abilities but each of us sees the world somewhat differently and interacts with others. Children benefit from the discovery of this basic fact — and parents do likewise. Your baby sees the world with an underpinning temperament and personality. You may have a cranky child wailing pitifully in foreign arms, a sleepyhead, or a gregarious kid laughing and cooing at everyone. A one-size-fits-all solution to parenting will not work, particularly in babyhood. Temperament develops into behavioral traits, as babies become infants. Your kid may be shy, cautious and defensive, often absorbed by new experiences in his own activities and hesitating about them. Easy, even-tempered types adapt to most situations more readily, while high-spirited infants tend to dive first in the head.

The Shy Child

This world's introverts can suffer more than most, and that can be particularly true in childhood. We have all seen the crazy mom driving her daughter into games at a party or the dad in the park forcing his timid son to the peak of a jungle gymnasium. If instead we recognize and validate how a child feels, it sends the message that it is okay to be who he is: "I know you don't like those horses on the carousel, Jack. You may want to try them out when you are bigger. "When a situation might be taxing a child, lay the foundation with quiet conversations:" We are going to a party for Grandpa's 70th birthday. There will be your cousins and aunts and uncles and those you do not know. Where do you want us to be when we chant Happy Birthday? "Note, too, that kids often shock us with an answer that we wouldn't have foreseen. A typical example is the child who hesitates with strangers and new situations but goes off to school in Montessori, and cannot wait to get back to school every morning after a day. What do us simply by conducting those challenges? Does that push our buttons? Particularly serious? None functions, and have we tried all the normal stuff? The first question to ask is whether that behavior is normal for the generation. Toddlers have limited spans of attention and poor social skills and are inclined to throw things out and explore beyond their own safety limits. Balancing their actions is often a question of managing your own aspirations: avoiding high-end restaurants, tracking situations that trigger tannery, giving a boisterous kid to let off steam, and seeking discreet corners for an anxious child in busy places. When you look at the situation, is it common behavior? When there is a new baby in the house, attention is often in short supply for the older child. "That's a beautiful new baby sister," her truculent grandson told a grandmother. "But now I want to read a story to someone who can talk to me." When all the families are in our house for the holidays or a family reunion, we might shortly see unrecognizable characteristics in an enthusiastic community of over-stimulated people, and we are making allowances. That said, some kids seem to pitch in every situation headlong, and there are times when it feels like their behavior is beyond control. Such a child needs regular ground rules reminders: you may not injure or harm yourself, other persons, or living things, nor may you intentionally damage the environment, be it your own possessions or other people's clothes. This kid needs to be given outdoor activities in all kinds of weather, with lots of interesting indoor hobbies. Challenging kids often come to expect negative reactions so notice good words and deeds and reward them. Remember that children evolve when they grow up, and when they are young what you consider intimidating can turn into positive characteristics when they get older. Children amaze us, right from the start they are men. We miss often.

Preventing Issues with Behavior

Prevention is better than cure, hence learning how to prevent problems with the behavior of children seems far better than learning what to do when you have a problem. Prevention has two main components: trying to learn to anticipate the behavior of your children; Work out how to prevent the possible issue.

Expectation includes learning by watching him about your child's behavior. See just how he plays with any toy, and how long he might last. What drives him into handling objects and playing with them? Are they giggling? Are those new ones? Require your guidance and support to make him play? Does he become frustrated by his incapability to do anything? Try breaking things, and taking them apart? How fast does he become bored? Observe how he responds in different situations: in the grocery store, in the house of another. Even before you understand how your kid is going to behave, you can begin anticipating what will occur and you will be ready. Anticipation is also assisted through constant monitoring of your preschooler. If he has been out of your eyes for ten minutes then he is probable to be exploring and is likely to get into trouble. The common lack of child monitoring (Patterson, 1982) is among the most notable characteristics of families where kids have the most difficult behavioral issues. So keep a close eye on the child all the way. If you cannot watch him then make sure, your spouse knows they have the responsibility to monitor him. It can be very exhausting because you feel you have to have eyeballs in the back of the head so you never feel you can concentrate completely on anything. That's why having your first child can be so exhausting because the older child will often disclose to you when you have more than one if the kid does something he shouldn't do. Just use the knowledge you gained by having watched your child and awareness of his or her developmental stage to prevent issues. Make the home environment safe, start by removing from the floor plants and electronic devices once your baby crawls. Use stair gates to stop him from going up and down the stairs when you do not look. Put child-resistant locks on kitchen cabinets. If your child gets bored sitting in the stroller, have toys and meals and drinks to use as interruptions if you are out of the home. Talk to him to get him involved in your activities; sing a song to get him involved and keep him happy; Go to the grocery store, which shows no sweets. Keep trips brief and do not expect him to sit gladly in the buggy for an hour while you are watching dresses.

There is an old study about watching mothers in supermarkets with their kindergartners (Holden, 1983). It showed that three different types of mothers. Some moms would scream at their kids and tell them off when they began misbehaving. The second group would divert the attention of their kids once they got tough. While the third group would escape problems, talking to their kids and getting them involved in shopping. The least problem had been for the mothers who could foresee the issues and reduce them before they even started. However, the moms who hollered had the hardest time and their kids made the most requirements on them. This study helps us to recognize how parenting style has a significant impact on the behavior of children. Their training is quick and your kid should be well conscious that if this is a diversion strategy that you used previously, you have everything in your pocket for him. He will scream and desire candy and biscuits if you have previously quieted him with all those. If he believes he can get you to start chasing him down and have a game, he will runoff. Therefore, if you see shopping as part of a social venture your kid is interested in, rather than waiting passively as you are moving home, you will notice he will be quieter for longer. He will eventually get bored, of course, as he does not want to look at the things you would like to look at; but you can purchase yourself for some time without crying and whining. This is a strong positive method of parenting, as it provides a strong relationship between your child and you. You think about the needs and interests of your child while doing what you wish to do as well. He starts to feel involved and appreciates chatting and attention. He is trying to notice stuff around him. You can direct his interest, broaden his language skills, and provide experiences of learning. For instance, enabling him to start putting the fruits and vegetables in the supermarket bags results in having to touch and feeling those foods. He learns their initials, feel, and smell. He also gets to practice counting. Having a chat like this can be hard work, and sometimes you feel a total idiot when you have been talking to the kid for the most part of the day and when he comes home, carry it on with your partner. This may be an important difference between men and women as women generally find it easier to chat about what they are doing, as opposed to giving a momentous commentary on their activities and emotions, whereas men tend to be silent and not verbalize their thoughts to the same degree. To reap the benefits of it, as it will only benefit your toddler.

Using Encouragement Instead Of Rewarding or Praising

Rudolph Dreikurs, an Adlerian inspired psychologist and author of Boys: The Task, said, "Kids require motivation as a plant needs water." Encouragement is a method of expressing the kind of affection that transmits to children that they are strong enough in their own way. Encouragement teaches kids that what they do is distinct from who they are. Encouragement lets kids know they are valued for their uniqueness without judgment. Through promoting, you show kids that errors are actually opportunities to improve and develop, rather than something they should be embarrassed about. Kids who feel motivated have a feeling of self-love and of belonging.

There is a contrast between appreciation and motivation. It is easy to praise or reward children who do well, but what can you say to children who have misbehavior and who don't feel good about themselves — when they need the most encouragement? "I have faith in you to handle this." "You're such a good problem-solver, I 'm sure you can figure out a way to solve this." "I love you no matter what." Praise and incentives teach children to focus on others' external decisions rather than following their own inner wisdom and self-reflection. So Instead of this example of praise: "I'm so proud of you," try encouragement: "You have to be very proud of yourself." Praise: "You've got an 'A.' I'll give you a reward." Encouragement: "You've worked really hard. You merit the 'A'

If your kid is over three, he will be able to understand the idea of receiving a reward. You should inform him that after you have said goodnight, you want him to sit in his bed or bedroom and if he does not come out, he will get a little surprise in the morning. This will function if your child is already willing to remain nights in his house, but not all. It means he has a chance to earn a reward. The present should be very small, for example on a chart, collector's cards, a crayon or a sticker. Do make a big fuss of what a clever boy he has been and how appreciative you are of him when you give it to him in the morning.

A healthy serving of praise and rewards motivates children to believe that "I'm all right only when others say I'm all right." It also tries to teach them to avoid mistakes rather than to learn from their mistakes. On the other hand, encouragement teaches them to believe in themselves, and their ability to do the correct thing. You should compose the inspiring notes to your family. People in some families turn up watching to encourage things to say and do for each other. Getting one complement ready for other family members once or twice a week may also be their task. Encouragement goes a long way to creating a healthy environment for the kids.

Better Self-Confidence and Self-Esteem for your Child

Ideally, we want our kids to grow up enjoying life, feeling about themselves, to be capable of dealing with their own emotions, and to be able to empathize with the feelings of others. We live in a competitive environment and some parents may think emotional tolerance is the reverse of the vigorously skills associated needed for success. However, it is not always achievable to be top of that list and most of the time we have to deal with being down a bit but feel Comfortable with the situation. Try to remember a many-year-old Charlie Brown children's show when Charlie decided to enter a school spelling competition and he did very well and did manage to get to the finals. Unfortunately, he fell by one point in the final round and became utterly despondent and feeling a complete loss. He had not appreciated having tried his best and done extremely well even though he had not come to the top. Helping kids feel confident about themselves is another way to inoculate them from bumps them will get all their lives. They are all always geniuses so there will still be somebody at school who considers the work harder or receives better grades. To avoid giving up on the competition and saying it is all a wastage of time, we need to help our kids feel proud of their achievements and efforts. Most schools now have 'Effort' grades on school reports, and those are more important than the 'Achievement' grade. The children who have low self-esteem tend to believe stuff is too difficult for them to do. They avoid being challenged, as they assume they will underperform. They can feel nervous or stressed and are easily hindered. They may then seek a lot of validation, take ages to get anything going, be very hesitant, and need encouragement repeatedly. In the preschool years, self-esteem and self-confidence begin. A child whose art efforts are giggled at or transformed upside-down and inquired, "What is that?" He is hi going to feel ashamed and start hiding his work, tearing it up, saying 'it's not good,' or stop doing it. Putting the artistic effort of your child on the fridge, empowering him to talk about what he is done in the picture, pointing out nice parts, and saying what a wonderful painter he is going to be producing a completely different set of feelings in him. He is more apt to seek again, make his attempts stronger, and feel able to show you what he had done. Your comfort and care as a mother or father are the most significant features of your children developing good self-esteem. Your constant and close connection is an essential cornerstone of how you perceive yourself and how you value yourself. The way they learn to respect themselves represents the opinion in them. Think about the people you meet, and how they think of their childhoods, about how they were handled by their parents. Many people would be explaining the strong expectations their parents have which they could never meet. They never felt that they were good enough for what they achieved. Sometimes this criticism is internalized and reappears when they are parents and suddenly they find themselves generating the same requirements for their children.

How to Make Your Children Listen to You

Do not pile any outage under the blanket of "not aware." Step in and find out what's really happening on, and then you can make an implementation plan to specifically address that issue. Therefore, if it is really a classic case of not hearing, here are seven steps you can take to make sure your kids understand you correctly.

1. Get to your point

Make sure you have her focus when you need your child's attention – that means eye contact. You not only validate that she sees and hears you as you lower yourself down and take a look at her in the eye, but you also strengthen communication. This suggests that you may need to step away from the washing or put the whisk down for a minute and walk into the other room. Proximity is key – you do not talk down to her or bark commands from the other room – you talk to her.

2. Do Not Get Away With "No"

Do not touch your dad. Do not run around in the hall. Do not just play with rice. Do not read out the following sentence. (Look what I have accomplished there?)

Negative orders like "don't" and "no" demand that children double the operation. There are two questions, which children will answer:

1) She does not like me to do what?

2) She needs me to do something instead.

That is humiliating and confusing. When you suggest, for example, "Don't touch your brother," a child will avoid the current behavior & decide the correct alternate conduct – when I can't reach him, does that imply I can't hug him? Can we match the tag? May I place a high five on him? Can I assist him to put his jacket on, or tie his shoes when asked by mom? Teach your kids what to do, instead. Try "Use gentle touches when touching your brother" or "Your brother doesn't like to be touched right now, so kindly keep your hands away while we are in the vehicle." Instead of "Don't leave your gadgets all over the mat," try "Please put your toys in the toy bin." rather than "Don't run in the hall," attempt "Please stroll in the hall."

3. Say Yes

Now think of it for a second. What is your natural, automatic response to your child's 5000 requests per day? "Yes," no?

It's hard to sift through them in a substantive way when you're overwhelmed by questions and you're only providing predetermined answers–" Sorry, not today." "Yes, I don't have room for that." "Sorry." "Nah, mate." "Nada.

However, if "no" is your perpetual go-to answer, it is no surprise children stop listening to your demands! Find reasons to say a more frequent yes. Your "yeah" responses will continue to confuse and delight your kids, and be more vigilant when you ask for something! Say, "The Park sounds great instead of" Sorry we cannot go to the beach! Was it Thursday after school or Sunday morning that we will go? "Instead of" Oh, oh ice cream "try" Ice cream is wonderful! Do you want to serve that Saturday or Sunday evening for dessert? "Although there will always be circumstances that require a strong 'no,' giving more 'yes' will improve your kid's odds of turning you back in.

4. Shorten the Conversation

Ah, child, I have been as guilty as anybody else in this has. Family, and particularly moms, tend to transform a short, quick five-second answer into some kind of five-minute-long study! Within the advertising business, there is a phrase, "Never market with blah-blah anything you will do with blah." I guess parenting makes sense, too. Be as descriptive as practicable when attempting to catch your kid's focus so they are not going to have room to shut you out!

5. Say Thanks Ahead Of Time

Support your children to make the correct decision by leaping confidence. Your preemptive "Thank you for hanging your towel during your shower," would motivate your children to act properly, even more than, "I'd best not see your towel again on the tile! "People will generally live up to our expectations and yes, even children, if we positively handle them. Allowing them to realize, in time, that you are confident in them to do the best thing would foster clear lines of contact and improve the probability of achieving the mission.

6. Ensure Awareness

An easy approach to make sure that your kid understood you

and that she knows is to encourage her to clarify what you said again. Studies in the medical community have found that 40-80% of the knowledge doctors convey to patients is either overlooked or ignored (and note, these are the adults we are thinking about, not just kids). Doctors have started using the teach-back method to combat this misinterpretation, which calls on patients to "teach-back" to the doctor what therapy instructions they have just been given. This approach has been shown to improve the patients' retention of information significantly. With babies, the same method can be used effectively. When you have made eye contact, simplified your voice, and clarified precisely what your child wants to do, politely remind your child to clarify what they have just learned. You will see an immediate increase in connectivity and unity in your household by ensuring everybody is on the same page.

7. Only make an assumption

When you see a job left unfinished, do not plunge in with a major reprimand, just make an observation: "I see a jacket on the deck," or you may say, "What's your intention today to take care of the trash? "For what end is your plan? "This is one of my favorites to stop political disputes. It is motivating as it is hypothesizing for your part that they have a strategy –

which offers your kid and chance to save face, which easily comes up with a solution in the moment they do not have one already! "Yeah, Yeah! I planned to take out the garbage right after I finished my lunch. "This gives you the opportunity to spin the whole conversation on a beneficial parenting empowerment spin! "That is great – I really appreciate your support, buddy.

Know, "not aware" is still a wake-up call for us. While on their part it may sound like provocation or inattention – it is more than probably a way to get our focus or show a desire for power. Children and adults alike deserve to be understood and observed. If the need is not fulfilled, children will avoid listening to us. It could sound perplexing, but it works simply because it is on the top of the list of complains parents share.

Being a parent can be full of problems and hardships. Keeping a balance for yourself and your partner is important. Your own emotional condition can have a huge effect on the emotional condition of your child and on his or her actions, and you ought to be mindful of how to remain calm and in contact with your emotions without getting upset. You will be better able to handle your kids, if you know yourself and follow the above given techniques and tips.

Conclusion

You will find realistic tips to improve your parenting knowledge by reading Toddler Discipline. Not only will you learn what isn't working, but what else can you do beyond it. You will discover new ways to motivate your kids to collaborate and excel without needing to use techniques of intimidation. Today the children need not be inspired by the fear of punishment. They have the inherent desire to realize what is right and wrong when given a chance to improve that skill. Instead of being inspired by punishment or intimidation, reward and the natural, healthy desire to please their parents can be easily motivated to them.

You will be introduced to basic infant problems, the Montessori Method of Learning, and will understand the different skills of parenting in the last two chapters of Toddler Discipline to improve communication, increase cooperation and motivate your children to be all they can be. In the last chapters, you will also figure out how to communicate the few most important things your kids need to hear repeatedly, which include:

- Being special is fine.

- Having errors is Fine.

- It is all right to tell no, but know the supervisors are mum and dad.

These messages will set your kids free to develop the abilities that God has given them. When well trained in the various techniques of constructive parenting, your child can acquire the qualities required to make a good life. Many of these qualities are empathy of others and oneself, generosity, deferred gratification, self-esteem, tolerance, resilience, consideration for others and oneself, collaboration, humility, honesty, and the capacity to be glad. Through the modern method mentioned in this book, your children will have the potential, along with your encouragement and help, to truly evolve at will period of their development. With such latest ideas, you will have the faith you need to get your kids up early and sleep soundly at night. When doubts and uncertainty emerge, you will have a strong tool to turn back to repeatedly to help you and reassure you of what your kids need and what you can do for them.

References

1. The Ages and Stages of Child Development. Retrieved from: **https://childdevelopmentinfo.com/ages-stages/#gs.75m6op**

2. The Montessori Teacher & Her Role. Retrieved from: **https://montessoritraining.blogspot.com/2007/09/montessori-teacher-and-her-role.html**

3. Montessori At Home. Retrieved from: **https://sapientiamontessori.com/montessori/montessori-at-home/**

4. Positive Parenting. Retrieved from: **https://www.cdc.gov/ncbddd/childdevelopment/positiveparenting/preschoolers.html**

5. How to Discipline Your Child. Retrieved from: **https://www.positiveparentingsolutions.com/parenting/how-to-discipline-your-child**

6. How to Get Kids to Listen. Retrieved from: **https://www.positiveparentingsolutions.com/parenting/get-kids-to-listen**

7. French Parenting. Retrieved from: **https://www.mydomaine.com/french-parenting**

8. What is Positive Parenting? Does it work? Retrieved from: https://www.positiveparentingsolutions.com/parenting/what-is-positive-parenting

9. How to Set Up a Montessori Space At Home. Retrieved from: https://livingmontessorinow.com/how-to-set-up-a-montessori-space-at-home/

10. Discipline and Guiding Behavior. Retrieved from: https://raisingchildren.net.au/toddlers/behaviour/discipline/discipline-strategies

PART 2

Positive Discipline

Introduction

Respect is among the most significant characteristics parents can help create in their children. Simple manners and respectfulness are critical for creating healthy relationships and for developing strong self-esteem. Unfortunately, because we reside in a digital world in which a culture of disobedience often dominates, it can be a difficult task to foster respect in our kids.

Is your kid disrespectful? Don't let the poor mood fall down on you! These suggestions can help set up a new environment in which respect is the law and not the exception.

My greatest belief in parental involvement is that the home of our family sets the backbone for the useful skills, characteristics, and lessons that we want to instill in our kids.

Kids, also young infants, recognize and try to mimic all we do. I would like to think of the home as the first school for our boy. So, let us just take the lead from traditional schooling, where teachers schedule and organize classes and set their students ' academic objectives. What do you want to know about your valuable kids? Most mother and father aspire to teach their kids how to be compassionate, honest, trustworthy, and considerate human beings who will end up making a positive impact in the world.

When you build your family's caring home base, they immediately obtain a lifetime gift — a safe sanctuary that safeguards them and enables them to develop, learn, enjoy, thrive, and acquire a positive sense of self. This secure, growing environment also allows people to make mistakes without the dread of feeling like a failure (usually plenty!). Rather, they can understand from their decisions and keep growing and flourish.

When our children are in a nurturing environment surrounded by a consistent dose of affection and learnable moments, they easily build a strategic sense of self-respect and respect for others.

• Teach homemade respect

• Help your child develop a sense of self-respect by taking care of themselves

• Be an emotional, healthy environment for your kid

• Demonstrate key social engagement skills to your kid

• Create a shared spirit

• Learn to speak a respectful language

Respect towards others coincides with the way that we behave towards ourselves. People radiating high self-esteem are powerful, healthy, positive humans who enjoy life with unbelievable vim and vigor. Opposite those with a confident sense of self are negative types that project doom and gloom on a regular basis.

Encouraging her to take care of herself is an easy and crucial way of teaching your child about self-respect. Staying alive improves our energy production, helps us to live in a more constructive frame of mind, and eventually encourages one to view the universe and others in a better way.

Taking care of oneself includes eating a healthful food and lifestyle routine, trying to keep up with personal care and hygiene, getting regular time to connect with oneself through reading, listening to songs, unplugging for an hour and enjoying with our thought processes, journalizing dreams, and aspirations — whatever motivates lifelong self-care.

Equally crucial for your child is building an emotional support system. Your actions and your way of talking to your child have a significant impact on the emotional safety of your child. Children view a scenario as unsafe when adults lift their tone, mark them, or call their names, equate one child to another, inflict drastic repercussions, or discipline them physically.

Chapter 1: Growth of babies (Birth to 18 months)

Your child's born and healthy. After a few months of exploration, worrying and hoping, the sweet scent of adorability is in your hands.

You do not want your baby to be with a conehead, but it does make total sense after its long stay in your busy and washing uterus, along with a tight grip through your birth canal. Luckily, she is amazing, and hoped that she will look better as the week progresses.

Seek to taste all the first bowls and kisses, first foods and skin snuggles. Now is the time for the process of your latest member of your family to begin. Remember that certain feelings of love and devotion do not always arise immediately, but rather it takes time to evolve within the coming weeks and months.

Where do you want to do this in the first birth week? Here's a glimpse.

1.1 The Infant Is 1 Week Old And Premature

This week, what is your baby going to do? She might lift her head slightly until placed on her tummy. You will also concentrate on items between 8 and 15 inches – the size of your face as you look at her, which you will be doing a lot of this week (and in the next weeks)!

But the main thing about their baby's behaviors may be those built-in reflexes in which all babies are usually affected, such as the very-important rooting reflex (when their faces are stroked, they shift in this direction) that lets the child find the nipple or the bottle, and the sucking reflex.

At first don't be fooled, because the girl seems sleepy. On the second and even third day of life a long period of marked drowsiness is expected — and presumably aimed at providing newborns with a chance to recover from their exhausting job (and you thought you were the only person who was tired!). When the weeks go on, her alertness will be higher. Take advantage of your sleepiness for now and chill while you sleep.

Your pregnancy and 1-week old infant growth

The baby weighs roughly 71/2 lbs and has a length of approximately twenty inches. Is your child larger or smaller? The vast majority of newborns in full term weight between 5 1/2 and 9 1/2 pounds between about Eighteen and twenty-two centimeters.

That is what you do not expect: your child will possibly lose some weight in the first few days after conception. In reality, nearly all newborns will leave their nursing home or childcare center as they check in for the first time with an expected loss of 5 to 10 percent of their birth weight during their first week.

Wondering whether your little one can regain weight? Breast-feeding babies — who only eat tsp of colostrums during their early eating days, don't get up well into their two-week birth weight. Babies fed the formula will see their excess weight gain more rapidly.

1.2 The Growth Of Your 2-Week-Old Infant

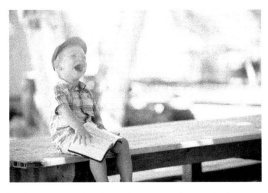

It does not feel like your kid is doing a lot of things these days — besides drinking, sleeping, and snacking. Yet she still utilizes a lot of her baby brain, alternating from observing closely what's happening (called the silent warning mode), running constantly, and sometimes creating tiny noises (called the aggressive alarm mode). She is still moaning, resting (either in silent sleep mode or active sleep mode), and spending time in a relaxed period (when the kid is just going to sleep or only waking up). Monitor closely, and you'll be able to adapt to the various states of mind of your baby over time.

While your baby looks like a fragile infant, with her beautiful little eyes, she is taking plenty of cognitive strides this week, like being able to concentrate on a name. And thinking of those lips, it is too early to say for certain what colour they are going to end up being. Many light-skinned babies are delivered with sky blue or slate-coloured eyes, while the remainder of babies with dark brown eyes appear. But the true colour of a baby's eye typically does not become completely understood until anywhere between 6 and 9 months, which will begin to shift as late as the first birthday.

Your rising 2-week-old infant

Starting next week, you will start writing bulletins for such weight gain. Many babies should have reached or exceeded their birth weight around 10 to 14 days of existence due to all the breastfeeding they do — whether from the breast or from the bottle.

Many babies in the breastfeeding division who get off to a late start can take a little longer to start piling on the pounds, so as long as the baby's doctor isn't concerned, you shouldn't be either. Only make sure the little one is feeding every two or three hours.

1.3 Development And Discipline

Discipline is less about punishing actions, contrary to traditional parental standards, and more about teaching kids strategies that allow them to act as per developmentally reasonable requirements. In addition, the term "discipline" originates from the Latin term "discipline," meaning "teaching."

Teaching your kids to be healthy and to live up to standards will start at "age zero," as we suggest, and grow from there. This is how :

Months 0-3: Setting the base

Successful discipline depends on a warm, loving partnership between parent and child, according to The American Academy of Pediatrics and reputable parenting gurus. Alternatively, suggests the AAP, terror is the reason for positive conduct rather than rationality, moral accountability, certain people's knowledge, or authority value.

You will start developing the bond by nurturing him when he's tired, cleaning, or dressing him when he's damp or freezing, hugging him when he's sad, and engaging meaningfully with him.

Months 0-3 are the "the fourth trimester" — a time where the infant cannot be abused. Indeed, several experts reinforce this by saying that replying consistently to the needs of your baby during this stage will lay a foundation of confidence between you, which is a crucial component of effective discipline.

Although at this point, rigid routines are not advised, routines may be begun to build. Routines let kids learn what to do, and may alleviate behavioral issues along the way, such as resisting bedtime or stopping playtime. Routines can ensure the infant is well-nourished and healthy and may deter inappropriate behavior right when it begins as infants prefer to act out while they are hungry or exhausted.

Months: four-nine

In the emergence of spinning, picking, sitting, and walking, you may want to cover your risky earrings for now and make sure that your house is babyproof.

Your baby doesn't understand right and wrong at this stage; through his developing gross and fine motor skills, and the tactile stimulation of picking objects and placing them in his mouth, he clearly learns about the environment. This is not only natural but also vital to his success. Here are some ways for him to set limits without meddling with any of these complicated duties:

• Discourage — cut off chances to snatch or say something that you don't want him to do. Apart from baby proofing, turn to stud jewelry for a while and place the enticing things on high shelves like remotes. It aims to raise the time you need to implement these next tactics:

• Distract — Note your kid is not checking boundaries at this stage; he 's interested. If you see him moving for a floor lamp that he loves to shake, stop him by stating something like, "Hey, look what I've got here! "And then:

• Redirect — offer him a toy, or participate with him to sing or go out. Whether you have glasses he can't avoid taking, or he keeps wanting to place shoes in his mouth, it typically does the trick by merely giving him nicely, tongue-friendly toys as an option.

The baby will continue to recognize "no" from the sound in the voice as you tell it, at 6 months of age. It's a strong term when he's heading towards a risky scenario that will halt him in his path. However, many experts claim that using "no" too often can diminish its strength or even prohibit a sense of wonder. We suggest that he be reserved for moments of threat or action such as punching or scratching. An alternative would be: "Cause it's dirty, we don't play with trash. Let's find a toy instead that you can play with."

Note that you clarify the reasoning behind the law in the illustration above, which is a common habit among parents of authority.

Months 10-18: Missing & Rational Consequences

Enhanced memory, an appreciation of cause and effect, and intellectual interest are adding fresh barriers to behavior. A typical example of this is to dump food on the ground. Why are babies fond of flinging food? They 're smart, Recall. Watching a blueberry roll over the floor while a dish of applesauce splatters is exciting and enjoyable for them. They 're also focused on your reaction to it; they may love the attention if you laugh or get annoyed.

And what would a mom do on her feet with applesauce? One strategy is to disregard this completely. Ignoring activity (as long as it isn't dangerous) works well if the kids are hoping for a response from you.

If ignoring isn't the trick, try to tell him with an unsympathetic face: "We 're not throwing food. We eat food. "At this phase, the meaning is reinforced by motions (shaking your head while mimicking tossing food in the first phrase, nodding your head while imitating placing food in your mouth in the second).

If, after you have said this, he tries to throw his food, use a logical consequence (one that is clearly relevant to the actions): tell him that lunchtime is now over and take him out from his high chair. You can give him a softball and say, "This is for tossing." If you're concerned that he's hungry, try to give him a snack a bit later.

Repeat this cycle, if he drops meal at the next session.

About Time-Outs?

Experts who advocate proactive discipline strategies usually oppose time-outs at this point, claiming that children are not able to grasp them in the developmental context.

Don't forget to employ humor.

The actions of your child often isn't a funny matter, but understanding when to use laughter in punishment will help encourage him and disperse heightened anger.

1.4 Support The Kid In Bed

Some kids sleep considerably more as compared to others. Few have long stretches of sleep, many in fast bursts. Some will sleep all night early, and others do not sleep long.

Your kid will possess its own awake and falling asleep pattern, and it's doubtful to be much like other newborns.

It's not even going to tie in with your sleep schedule. Take naps while your child is sleeping.

Your kid would definitely doze off after a feed for brief amounts of time if you're breastfeeding, in the early weeks. Start feeding before your kid is done, or when they're completely asleep. It is a perfect time to seek to give yourself a little relaxation.

If you don't sleep together with your kid, don't think about holding the house quiet when they're sleeping. It is important to have the baby accustomed to sleeping with any noise.

Get your kid accustomed to day and night?

Teaching your kid regarding night-time being separate from daytime during the start is a smart idea. Open curtains throughout the day, play games, and while they sleep, don't think a lot about daily sounds.

In the evening you can find it beneficial to:

• Keep your lights low

• Don't talk too often and hold your speech steady

• Lay the kid down until they are fed and cleaned

• Do not modify your kid unless they require it

• Don't interact with the kid

Gradually the kid must know that the time of night is for bed.

Where to sleep, my baby?

Your child should be in the same location as you during the initial six months, day and night, because they're asleep. Particularly in the early days, you can find your baby is always sleeping in your partner's arms, or when you're sitting by the cot.

You will begin to have your baby habituated to sleep by providing them comfort by having set them down until they go to sleep or after a meal has just ended. This may be more complicated to achieve if your child continues to be alert more frequently or for longer.

Asleep Newborn: what to anticipate

Newborn kids sleep all day, through the night, on and off. It may be helpful to have a timetable but you can also tailor the procedure to your desires.

For example , right before you head to bed, you could decide to wake the kid up for a feed in the expectation you'll have a decent night's sleep before they wake up in the morning.

Establishing a child's sleep schedule

When your child is about 3 months old, you can be ready to implement a sleep schedule. Having them into an easy, comforting sleep schedule can be easy for everyone, and help avoid later sleep issues. It's can also be a perfect chance for your kid to have face to face attention.

the schedule consists of:

• Taking a shower

• Changing between nightwear and a new nappy

• Laying them down to rest

• reading stories at bedtime

• Dim the lighting inside the room to build a quiet ambiance

• Offering a cuddle and a good night hug

• Humming a love song or getting a magical wind-up screen you should toggle on when you place your child in bed

• brush their teeth (if any!)

When your child grows older, sticking to a consistent schedule in bedtime will be beneficial. Too much energy and noise will wake your kid up again, close to bedtime. Take considerable time calming down to do some relaxing things, such as meditation.

Give up a little room between feeding and going to bed for your infant. If you nurse your child to bed, both eating and sleeping would become linked inside your newborn's mind. So if they wake up during the night they might want a feed to assist them to return to nap.

How much the child needs to sleep?

Just like adults, sleep patterns for babies and kids vary. Some kids have had somewhat more or less sleep from birth than others.

Newborn's sleep requirements

Most newborns are more dormant than awake. Their average cumulative sleep differs but may be between eight hours and sixteen or eighteen hours. During the evening, babies wake up as they have to be fed. Staying too cold or hot will interrupt the sleep, too.

Sleep criteria at ages 3 to 6 months

As your child grows, they will need lesser night-time feedings and can sleep longer. Few babies will cycle every night for eight hours or longer, but not all. By 4 months, they can spend about twice as much night sleep as they do throughout the day.

Sleeping at 6 to 12 months

Night feeding may no longer be needed for babies between six months to a year, and some babies can nap for 11 hours at night. Any babies can wake up in the night with teething pain or starvation.

Sleeping criteria at twelve months

After their first birthday, babies will sleep for twelve to fifteen hours.

Two-year-olds requirements for sleep

Most of the 2-year-olds sleep at night for eleven to twelve hours, with 1 to 2 naps during the afternoon.

Sleeping needs for 3 to 4-year-olds

Most kids aged 3 or 4 will need approximately twelve hours of sleep, but that can range from eight to fourteen hours. During the day, other little children would always require a break.

1.5 Tackling Infant Sleep Issues

All kids alter habits during nights. When you feel you've figured things out and you've both had a decent night's sleep, you could get up every three hours the next night.

Be ready to adjust habits as the kid develops and moves through various stages. And note, spurts of development, teething, and diseases will all influence how your kids to sleep.

Whether your kid has sleeping issues, if you need some advice about settling into a schedule, chat to your health visitor.

Chapter 2: Toddlers (18 months to 3 years)

Expect rough phases. Many of the day's circumstances and moments seem to cause negative conduct. Main suspect number 1: moves from one task to another (waking up, heading to bed, leaving playing to have dinner). Giving your kid a heads-up, and he's more positioned to turn modes ("We'll have dinner after you construct that block tower"). Select your wars. When you tell no 20 times a day, it's going to lose its impact. Prioritize habits into a major, small, and negligible ones to mess with. There are screw-ups in Venti, Grande, and Tall Toddler in Starbucks terminology. If you overlook a small crime — your kid cries while you read your inbox — she'll finally quit doing it, and she'll know it's not having a raise from you.

2.1 Development And Discipline

• Use defense. Sorry for the cliché of football, but this one is simple. Render your house child-friendly, and hope fairly. When you clean off the end table, your selection of Swarovski crystal, your kid would not be compelled to fling it on the TV screen. When you're getting dinner with your mates, go early, and you're not going to have to queue for a seat.

• Quick and nice statements. Speak in brief sentences such as "No striking." This is far more efficient than "Chaz, you know it's not good to hit the pet." You'll lose Chaz immediately after, "you know."

• Bring forward the effects. Your child will understand its normal behavioral consequences — better recognized as action and reaction. Of, e.g., if he insists loudly on picking his pajamas (that takes an extended period of time), then he always prefers not to read books until bedtime. Trigger: Extended pajama-picking = impact: No chance for reading. He may select his pj's faster next time, or let you select them out.

• Don't hide to prevent confrontation. We always want to be the party pooper, so even to avoid a confrontation at the grocery store, you shouldn't give in. When you believe your kid can't have the food she saw on television, hold to your weapons. You'll be glad to have done that eventually.

• Pay heed to offers. Sure, when your focus is distracted, your little angel can behave up (making dinner, chatting on the phone). That's why giving some amusement (a beloved toy, a speedy snack) is essential. Real fact: My son consumed pet food once, when I was with a customer on the line. Take-home lecture: When you don't give your baby anything to do while you're distracted, she'll find it — and it may not be a nice performance.

• focus on observable, not on the boy. Often claim there's poor stuff like that. Never tell your kid how poor he is. You want him to think you respect him, but the way he is behaving right now, you don't respect him.

• Offer kids options. It should help her feel like she has a choice. Just make sure you're not giving so many choices because they're just items you intend to do, like, "It's your decision: you can wear your shoes first, or your jacket first."

• Do not shout. But it does shift the voice. It's not the quantity that gets your argument across but your tone. Recall The Godfather movie? Don Corleone has never had to shout.

• Catch good to your boy. If you compliment your kid when he does a positive attitude, he will do so more frequently — so he will be less inclined to act poorly only to gain your focus. The Reward system for that superego is fertilizer.

• Respond right away. Don't wait to have your kid punished. She won't know that she's more than five minutes into trouble until she's performed the dirty deed.

2.2 Toddler Testing Behaviors

Situation #1:

Your 18-month-old spends most of your game group session climbing and wriggling on your lap, using you as you sit on the floor to pull up to standing.

Parents may not realize this conduct as a test because a) It usually starts early in the infancy when we are habituated to respond to the more straightforward behavior of our infant (child demonstrates a need, we perceive it and try to fill it); b) we may not be affected by this conduct while our baby is small; c) we may even think it's a good thing to let babies jump on us.

A child who is mature enough to squirm, jump, cling and climb is also mature enough to realize that "I love to have you on my lap, but I need you to rest still. You should use the coffee table (or whatever) whether you decide to crawl or pull up. "I guess kids need the boundary to be transparent, and they can make a safe choice to step away from the adult to remain near.

If the kid starts wiggling (which is likely to continue even if he actually knows our vocabulary – that's what monitoring is), we carry through: "I'm going to push you off my arm, since you're having difficulty staying still. You want to climb on me. This makes me feel uncomfortable.'

The secret to knowing the difference between a need and a desire is the key. There might well be a need for closeness and contact in the play-on-the-lap case, but the use of mom or dad as a climbing mechanism is a wish and, more than possible, a check.

In this situation, the question the child asks, though not consciously, is, "How much will you let me do to you? "When parents authorize this test to go, even though they are upset or irritated, even if they are not sure, it will become the subject of the child (as other assessments do).

I would always allow a child to stay in my lap (without squirming) as long as he wants, in a playgroup or other social setting (and even during playtime together at home). I strongly recommend staying in these environments so that kids have opportunities to build trust as free explorers, deciding autonomously when to return back to their parents (referred to as their "secure base" by attachment theorists Bowlby and Ainsworth).

Instead, I do not advocate coaxing kids to let us "play over

there with all those fun things," or "see what Joey does," etc. Kids know when we sell them on something!

Situation #2:

Your 18-month-old is incapable of making up his mind. He chooses to go outside first. He wants to come back in two minutes later. He decides to head out again a minute later.

Toddlers want to determine. Or do they? They aren't very aware. The immature years are a period of contradictory, unbridled feelings sometimes articulated by impulsive, rebellious behavior.

I was interviewing a parent recently, whose three-year-old son was doing the reverse of everything she told him to do. If she said, "do not," she was able to count on him to do whatever it was instant. It made me chuckle when she provided that her noncommittal answers such as "either way is fine" would totally stop him in his paths because he couldn't think of an intolerable option to take. (She had given birth to a second child recently, and his analysis made a lot of sense.)

If we hear 'red,' toddlers have a rather powerful desire to utter 'blue,' and then if we decide to say 'blue,' there is a fair risk that they would have to switch back to 'no, red.'

To help extricate the children from these power and resistance cycles, they need us to gently make some of these choices for them, thus understanding their perspective. And we follow up by encouraging them to pursue our path.

In other terms, anytime a kid has a second (or maybe even the first) change of mind when it sounds irrational or unlikely, we reply, "I think you want to go outside. We're going to do that a little later after I've finished making your lunch. We are going to stay inside for now.

As normal, our positive disposition and complete tolerance of the adverse reaction of our child to our decisions are much more important than the language that we use.

2.3 Guide To Taming Tantrums

Around 85 percent of kids of 2- and 3-year have tantrums. According to the National Association of School Psychologists, they typically tend to appear while children are between the ages of 12 and 15 months, ranges between 18 and 36 months, and persist until about the age of 4.

Why is that? As one aspect, there is a shortage of physical, motor, and language abilities in young children to achieve what they desire and may contribute to anger, understandably. (How would you sound if you needed a knife, but couldn't touch the silverware cabinet, so everyone believed you were saying "stool?") As Dr. Daniel J. Siegel, a neuro-psychiatrist, wrote in his novel, "The Whole-Brain Baby," children in this age range, "haven't learned the opportunity to use language and vocabulary to convey their emotions, so they've failed to communicate their thoughts. That's why they tend to be oblivious of any health needs, propriety, punctuality, or any other justification you may have for asking any kid to quit or continue doing something.

In many parents, tantrums inspire anxiety. Enter in a search engine "how to handle tantrums," and you'll get hundreds of thousands of answers. This severity of parental concern makes sense, given how destabilizing the tantrums can be. Your most respectful, mostly well-behaved toddler becomes a monster out of nowhere, stomping and screaming if you don't meet his demands. Tantrums can also transform parents, causing us to say and do things that we will regret later, such as shouting — or, worse, caving into the demands of our children. But with a little careful planning, before they launch, you will learn how to fend off other tantrums and respond as gently and tactfully as possible when your kiddo melts down.

I discussed four child psychologists for this guide, along with many psychologist-approved manuals for general discipline and tantrum control. The overarching lesson is that tantrums, although stressful, are a natural part of infant growth — so preparing to handle them (when you can't avoid them) is an integral component to every parent's ability set.

Understand that tantrums are normal toddler behavior.

What causes tantrums

Many kids are more susceptible to tantrums, particularly ones who are violent, hyperactive, or moody, or those that are not well adjusted to new environments. Tantrums are clearly a means for most children to break rid of their agitation and check boundaries (will mommy give me the gift if I scream loud?).

The simplest items will set off little children from telling them to take a bath when they are in the midst of enjoying Sesame Street or requesting them to swap a beloved plush toy with a younger sibling. Any change-inducing condition will cause a tantrum. Apply exhaustion or hunger to the mix, and children become much more prone to throw a tantrum with their tolerance threshold even smaller.

Ensure your child is safe and, if necessary, move him.

This may seem evident, but if your child is at risk of endangering himself or others, or damaging property, move him somewhere safer, rapidly and calmly. When you're in a public setting — a shop, a restaurant, a church service — where a tantrum will be upsetting, the recommendation to move him still applies. "Yes, they might hit you or kick you," said Dr. Ellen Braaten, Ph.D., a psychologist, assistant professor at Harvard school of public health, and co-director of the Young Healthy Minds Clay Centre. "But remain true," Dr. Braaten said. "Do whatever easily takes you out, without getting upset."

When the child's in a healthy spot, you can seek certain ways of tantrum-taming.

Try to keep your calm

Here's some advice that Dr. Rebecca Schrag Hershberg, Ph.D., a professional psychologist and founder of "The Tantrum Survival Guide," has passed along: The thermostat is what a parent should be, not a thermometer. "The aim is to reset the temperature," she told me. "Don't take it and react to it." She clarified that if you're not relaxing down, it's even worse for the child to calm down. Dr. Hershberg recommended that you note that tantrums are not personal: it is not your fault that your kid has a tantrum, but it is your duty to help lead her out. Pause and give some caring reassurance for your kids. Take a deep breath. If it does support, count backward. If you have difficulty holding your composure, consider making a note of why you may be suffering. Possibilities include circumstances (for example, if your child throws a tantrum during a particularly stressful morning) or personal experiences ("Mom does not let me get away with that").

How to Stop the Screaming

The best approach to avert a temper tantrum is to offer what the kid needs. Obviously, in the long term, this tactic won't do you much good, since your kid will always go into tantrum mode if he needs something.

The first move in fighting a temper tantrum is to hold your own emotions under control. If both of you are yelling at each other, you won't get anywhere with your child. It's also not a safe idea to hit your kid, and it'll just make the tantrum worse. Take a deep breath, take hold of your feelings, and then punish your boy by letting him realize gently but clearly that tantrums are not appropriate behaviour.

If your kid is ever not able to settle down and you realize that the tantrum is just a trick to gain your focus, don't give in. Even if you have to drag your screaming kid through the supermarket, just ignore the tantrum. It's simpler to tell than shot, but hold to your guns, and hopefully, the lesson will be the period, and she'll realize you're sincere, and this won't work out. When your kid is convinced that the temper tantrum doesn't carry her anywhere, she'll quit screaming.

If your child is distressed to the extent of becoming devastated or out of balance, hug him firmly to comfort him. Tell him softly that you value him but don't offer him what he needs. If it doesn't succeed, push him out of the scenario and place him in a time-out for one to two minutes and allow him time to cool down. The general guideline for the duration of a time-out is one minute of the child's age each year.

Use every weapon in your arsenal

Much like every kid is special, so too is every tantrum. Because no one approach can avoid each tantrum any time with each kid, I suggest that you familiarize yourself with many specific methods of tantrum-taming. With experience, each of the following strategies should become easier and more efficient. So fear not — your child will certainly offer you lots of realistic opportunities.

Peacefully try to hug your kid. Please be sure, and this doesn't imply holding your kid physically or pushing him to hold you against his will. Yet an expression of your love and affection can reassure an overwhelmed child.

Try to distract. When your child's brother, for example, has grabbed his car, you may be willing to stop the tantrum by giving him another one. Certain ways of diversion worth exploring involve shifting the atmosphere by going to another space or having the favorite music of your child on. The technique of diversion appears to function best for younger children, whose perceptions are shorter and who may neglect their emotions from moment to moment.

Suggest methods of self-calming. It involves a little strategic preparation, although older children should be given methods such as taking calming breaths or counting backward, which can be remembered to pursue when a tantrum hits them.

Stop the tantrum. Please be sure, and this does not imply totally ignoring your child: you will remain in the space and be accessible physically and emotionally. Nonetheless, you should decline to indulge in the protests and yells, and then concentrate on supporting your child with an irrelevant need. "For example, if your child is crying and whining because they can't wear their favorite outfit, you can ignore that aspect of what they're saying and still look after them in other ways by, say, helping them get on their shoes." When your kid is always screaming, for example, but has avoided stomping her foot, thank her for that.

Time-out is a loaded word, but let's be specific on what this approach is not. It doesn't mean holding your child in the corner as punishment or taking him to his bed. The time-out solution to handling tantrum includes reminding the kid in a quiet voice that you're going to wait for her to cool down, and that you're looking forward to interacting again once this occurs. This approach is especially helpful when you feel frustrated yourself (you can also acknowledge that your child feels this as a means of showing empathy).

Try to reach the core of the problem

Tantrums are a form of expression. It's not that distinct from when your child was an infant, moaning because he was hungry or because he had a dirty diaper. What the kid is actually doing in a rant is attempting to express something to you in the best manner they can. The tantrum of your child may be a sign of hunger, tiredness, illness, or even disappointment that they don't get their way. Perhaps the underlying cause of a tantrum may be quickly detected and resolved — by, for example, having a minute to relax or getting a snack. More complicated are those tantrums that don't seem to represent a physical cause, tantrums that are sparked by sheer anger — at your cruel rejection to let your kid run on the street or play with the burgers. In these situations, start by voicing empathy towards your child (and maintaining her safety), then pass on to one of the below time-tested strategies.

2.4 Gaining Confidence As A Parent

I sit by the swimming pool on a sweltering Saturday afternoon, watching two boys play in the water. I see a little kid, clothed in a pink swimsuit, jumping back and forth into the water. Her father is poised to capture her. She squeals in amazement. She then leaps beyond his control, and there comes a look of fear across his face. He dashes in order to catch her just in time. Her smile is pure bliss- but one of fear and relief of her father.

The scene made me think of what it takes to develop parental trust. Trust is such an important part of parenting – so essential that it's hard to think about or describe it. What was it that allowed this little girl to trust her father and think he is trustworthy and will do the right thing?

How does emotional maturity help parents build confidence in their children? As we all know, confidence is built from the early years of childhood, beginning with a sequence of successful experiences between a parent and infant. Trust built by the bond between parent and child is transferable to other circumstances and has a profound effect on the willingness of one adult to communicate with others. Here are 10 practical tips for building confidence as a parent:

Trusting our emotions

Emotions (theirs and ours) can look big when our children are young. The major feelings can sometimes be destructive and even obstructive. Parents tend to feel stressed at juggling a lot of tasks against tight deadlines. And when kids throw tantrums and don't do what we expect of them, we generally have little patience to cope with these feelings, so our instinct is to rush through them with incentives, intimidation, and distractions. Yet to help our children develop self-confidence, we need to educate them about their feelings, and how feelings are responses about themselves. The first move is to increase their awareness regarding emotions.

Recognize your children's emotions by using the neutral language to describe what you observe: "I see you're very frustrated with your sister."

Help them mark their feelings and develop their emotional literacy gradually: "How would you explain what you feel right now?"

Validate the sentiment you see: "I can see that you're angry with your mate." Validating doesn't automatically imply you're in accordance with the thought. You're simply acknowledging it, so you should consider their viewpoint.

The theory behind this last suggestion is that as we affirm the feelings of our children, we allow them time to relax and be welcomed in the way they behave. Meanwhile, their amygdala can calm down, so we can then work with them to solve the issue.

Taking emotional responsibility:

At one point, when she was attempting to get out, the little girl hit her knee against the wall at the pool. She cried, but her father did not instantly come to her rescue. He let her sob as she kept going, all the while urging her to continue attempting. She'd made it over the building. She knows at this point that she might bring herself out of a poor situation. She's discovering that she can fix her own issues. The little girl is trying to support herself in this accident.

They are creating the foundations of a trustworthy partnership as they encourage children to take accountability for their own feelings. The principle of moral accountability is that each of us is liable for how we react and how we treat our stimuli.

Learning by demonstration is the perfect way to demonstrate the moral obligation. When you're in a confrontation with another human, let your kids see how you take moral accountability for the problem "behind the screen."

We can understand our choices better when we tune in and notice when we observe ourselves in action. Then we'll know the successful ones and others that aren't. Share your patterns with each other as a family, and ask what others are observing about yours.

Brainstorm ways each individual can assume responsibility for their patterns. Getting fully mindful about, and take accountability for, our thoughts will inform our children about meaningful thought.

2.5 Importance of Communication

Your kid isn't conditioned to neglect you — she's only studying words, and she can be baffled by what makes sense to you.

When you tell: "be quiet!"

You say that We are in the book store and I am shocked that you are so rude!

Why the baby doesn't understand it: Children must modify their voice in order to control the impact of impulses. "Besides that, social skills — including the ability to understand when a scenario advocates for a quiet voice — take patience for internalization.

Chat Baby Whisper: "Use your accent! "Young children are copycats by definition, so once you show the child how you would want him to communicate, Dr. Borba advises that he can really listen. Sometimes, at home, practice communicating in" silent voices." "This will make it simpler once you encourage the kid to move actions from a protected atmosphere to the practical world, face to face around you, "suggests Dr. Borba. Eventually, apply the principles of the particular setting with which he or she is in.

Saying: "Be gentle!"

You mean Stop Animal Torture!

For beginners, she may not realize what soft entails. On top of

that, infants are still developing empathy. While your kid may start realizing other people have feelings, she's still pretty egocentric — and she won't think about how her actions impact others all the time.

Inspire the little one to understand better by verbalizing love for her. You might suggest, "When you grab his tail, it really scares the cat — just as it feels when you fall down." Then attempt to offer a more precise order when you reach the correct way to do it to your child. Suggest "This is how we pet a kitty," for example, by taking her hand and using it to softly rub your pet. Say the term soft many times as you do so, demonstrating what it truly is. Finally, allow your kid the chance to do something by themselves. After saying 'nice' in emphasis when stroking the cat together, tell, 'You're showing me compassion now.

If you say: "Do not act rude!"

You want to say, Show me a bit of respect!

The reason, your baby, doesn't understand it: They tend to get resistant as small children know their style has energy. Toddlers speak back, so limits are being tested. They 're beginning to demand their rights; this is one path. And when you order her to place back her toys, if your kid starts

shouting "No!" it's not that she starts pretending to give you a tough time; extra control is what she is looking for.

Talk like a kid: You don't have to take it too seriously and shout at your baby when she acts difficult — it's a normal move to turn into an adult. The easiest way to connect is to pattern. Tell gently, 'It's not nice to speak to me in this way. First, encourage her with some deliverable choices. They may say, "Would you like to put back markers or books initially?" There are greater chances that she will comply if your child is given some of the power she's looking for.

When you tell: "If you repeat that, you'll be given timeout!"

Do you say you can't listen to orders and follow them?

Why not get it for your kid? Just after you made that threat, what precisely impacts your kid to do stuff again? Ok, it's not like he actively rejects you (you might later look into that!). "Even now, little kids have not acquired the ability to recognize action and reaction. In other terms, recommending the child that if he proceeds to do anything he is prevented from doing, there will be risks.

Do not talk! The best approach to solve the dilemma is to remove the kid entirely from the scenario and have him think about something else. Even if he doesn't avoid splashing the milk in the pet dish, turn his concentration back: take him up gently, move him to couch and initiate a new job together, like completing a puzzle.

The Moment you tell: "get inside the room and ponder over your actions!"

You imply I have to feel that you are dying in the guilt!

The reason your child won't realize that "that's like instructing the dog to recognize what he's executed. A kid who is 2 is almost as likely to take the route as a cat is! Many kids can't focus on what they've achieved in a constructive manner."

You can't really expect your child to consider about his own actions and realize the mistakes of his actions — instead you may assist him to find the exact way to behave. Dr. Holland says that as he learns the acts you like to do better by observing and behaving than by reacting to something you are lecturing on about what is right and what is wrong, consider posing and performing the roles. Of starters, if your kid fails to share toys and steal the toys of other siblings, make sure that he watches you share the pieces of apple with his elder bro at mealtime. When he gives you a piece, say a huge "thank you!" while you share a piece with him later. You can also arrange a cozy tea fun party with animals and make him experience doing it with them. If you're playing a good behavior session, he may want to jump in, of course.

2.6 Help Your Kid Start Talking

When your kid starts communicating, it's a whole new universe-and that's what they've been dreaming for all this long! Here are a few strategies to motivate your little one to get the vocabulary started, as a pediatric speech therapist has suggested. All the children are special, as you know, and they grow at their own rate. Consult a doctor if you have any worries regarding the development of your little one.

Use Sign Language

Child sign language has been shown to help kids grow better vocal competencies faster. It may seem counter-intuitive, but using symbols can help communicate with the little ones, and the enthusiasm they feel about that actively motivates them to talk.

Start with a couple of signs — start with the ones you would sometimes use with things like "more," "all done," and "baby"—and integrate them into your everyday routine. Always tell the phrase exactly as you do the symbol, and also repeat both the symbol and the term.

Reduce time in front of a screen

Children learn from having contact actively with their worlds, something which doesn't happen when parked in front of a

TV or laptop. And studies show that time on screen in children under the age of three is linked to delayed language development. For children two years old and older, the American Academy of Pediatrics suggests limiting the screen time to 2 hours a day. And younger children and infants should be hindered from playing with TVs or watching them at all.

Talk About Everything

Word-exposure is crucial when learning to speak a language. So talk — lots of it! -- To your baby. Use easy short words, talk calmly. Keep it communicative, listening to your kid, and letting him respond with plenty of stops and starts.

Can't think of a word? Just say what you are doing with your little one. While dining, pretend to be on a cooking show that explains how to make the food. Tell the names of the garments and what you're doing as you get your little clothed: Now, we're attempting to pull the T-shirt over your neck!

Be his sound

Repeat what your kid says to you, trying to add as you do,

with one or two words. Called echo expansion modeling, child speech therapists suggest this method to inspire children to further grow their expressive speech.

Don't assume

Make a tiny bit of your kid work for what it wants! Wait till he speaks, instead of predicting each need and appeal.

Challenge Jibberish

You have pretended for so long to comprehend baby talk, and it might function normally to respond to a nonsensical phrase. But if your kid is at the level where he can move beyond mumbling, it's smarter to let him understand you don't recognize what he's talking about. Tell him softly, "I liked you talking, but I'm sorry, I don't understand you.

Read

Books are a perfect way of introducing your kid to vocabulary and to grow a passion for reading that supports him throughout his life. Read every single day to your kid. You can also read all the road signs, the advertising copy on the cereal box, and the product names in the supermarket, aloud.

Encourage words

When your kid talks, be gracious and particular in your

admiration. For instance, if she asked by title for yogurt, tell her how happy you are of her use of the word for yogurt. It's a great time to share a few more words as well; you might add that yogurt is chilly and promotes good strong bones.

Be blind to signs

Your little one might be unwilling to work on her speech if he finds gestures that do the job just fine, thanks a lot. Delay your reaction to his actions to support his focus on words. If he points to inquire for more berries, just hesitate and see how you can make her spit the term out.

Make sure that you use the word repeatedly when you answer to his request and let him know what you're doing: "Do you want more apple? I'm very pleased to provide you with an apple. Those apples are crunchy and sweet! I also like them.

2.7 Why The Way You Talk To Your Child Matters

As parents, we care a lot about how our kids are relating to us and how they are acting. If they require correction, we'll warn them, and ensure they have proper manners to guide them away from bad conduct. Yet we may not always be careful of what we utter and how we utter it.

Consider how you communicate with your kid.

We also have trouble looking critically into our own behaviour. When you ponder how to explain how you communicate with your child on a regular basis, visualize capturing your experiences and bringing back recorded photos and sound. Does that sound gentle and caring for your voice? Do you want to be involved and active in what your child has been saying? Or can you see yourself phubbing your child (phone snubbing)—texting mates, reading mobile messages — instead of giving complete attention to your kid? In other terms, if you were filming yourself and playing it back, would you have felt you were at your strongest?

If the response is no, then ask what you might do to improve the way your child interacts. Was your voice stern, irritated, or frustrated as you speak to your kid about everything that she has done wrong? Do you sound like a cross with your mom, even though she did nothing improper because you are tired?

Think of the tone of voice you 're adopting and pay particular attention to how you should change it while you're talking about your kid, especially though a behaviour problem is being addressed.

Specific explanations of why expressions and sounds tend to be more optimistic

Below are a few significant explanations of why your voice tone and the phrases you use will make your parent-child contact and experiences even more constructive and gratifying:

Your kid would have a better likelihood of hearing. That's fundamental logic. What would you prefer — anyone who talks to you in a harsh or negative tone or someone who talks to you in a cool, fair, and sweet voice? And if there's a dispute or you need to fix something that your child does, a soft voice, even though it's stern, is going to attract more focus from your kid, so she'll be more inclined to listen to what you suggest.

You are going to have a better link. You will be reinforcing your relationship as you handle your kid with compassion and support. Say " thank you "and" please "when you talk to your kids and inform them clearly that you want him to do the same thing. You will get closer to each other by treating one another with good manners and respect; mean statements and a cruel voice will have the opposite effect.

Being stern doesn't work. If you call out to your child or act harshly, you are less apt to get positive outcomes, and could even damage your partnership. Nevertheless, evidence suggests that shouting may be as dangerous as a harsh discipline.1 The child might be attentive in the short term, but if you want the child to build the knowledge, he wants to control his own behaviour, communicating politely is obviously the safest path forward.

Children benefit from our actions. The easiest place to get your kid to speak to you politely is by talking to her kindly. Even if you attack her excessively, even talk negatively to her? Okay, you can say what you are going to get out of it.

Your child should kindly handle peers, teachers, and others throughout his life. If you adopt a good tone of voice for your kid at home, she'll do so in school and in other situations, of course. This will not be long until everyone around your kid remark about her good etiquette and sweet way of communicating, and she will be proud of those qualities that will bring her into puberty and beyond. Visualize it: a respectful teen who actually speaks out in a civilized manner! It is likely because you are already instilling these techniques.

2.8 Stop Your Child's Whining

Almost since my baby, Liz was able to talk in sentences, she

complained anytime she was not able to get what she was looking for: my love, a cookie, a repair job on a defective doll. After she turned 3--and immediately felt like a "big girl"— began to make me insane with her constant moaning, underneath my breath, I would mutter loudly, clench my jaw, even moan back. Once I lost composure and so loudly yelled, "shut up!" that she erupted into tears. Yet more frequently than not, just to make the whiny tone disappear should I let her have what she wanted.

As nails on a blackboard, whining — an annoying combination of speaking and crying — has the potential to make nearly any parent get upset or give in. Yet preschoolers are extremely intelligent: they realize their parents are heavily influenced by begging in the appeal.

Moreover, a whiny kid is not meant to be irritating or abused. Whining is also the only way small children will show themselves whether they are exhausted, cranky, thirsty, unhappy, or simply don't want to do anything. While the language abilities of 3- and 4-year-olds are growing quickly, they also may not have the vocabulary to express any of these emotions.

Punishment Can backfire

Even though your kid may express, for example, that she is starving for lunch or that she hates staying in her car seat, she may always complain as she has understood by practice that you should be paying attention to this attitude. "Whining helps them feel really strong with children exploring the boundaries of their freedom.

"If you can't bear crying, your kid can do it even more, just because it creates a response," says Jane Nelsen, Ed. D., co-author of Constructive Reinforcement for Preschoolers. They 're likely to go for a pessimistic response because they don't understand how to get a better answer, "notes Nelsen. So needless to say, give in (Okay, you may have one slice of candy but guarantee you'll have your lunch? You 're not going to succeed either. You 're going to get a moaning respite, yet you're always propagating the issue.

Luckily, you can interrupt this cycle — in a manner that facilitates the growth of your kid rather than punishing her. "If you avoid being irritated with the moaning, your kid should quit too," Nelsen maintains. At first, this laissez-faire method seems to be entirely impractical, but as my daughter was a whining lover, I wanted to seek it out.

This wasn't easy — often, I was inclined to yell or simply give

her whatever she wanted — but I was resolved to remain strong and persistent. "You have to show a lot of self-control," says Dr. Crowder. To my astonishment, after a matter of weeks, Elizabeth had settled into the routine of demanding politely rather than nagging.

Steps to Habit Breaking

Give recognition where appreciation is due. "Parents often find out, 'That's not a good sound,' but sometimes don't have enough constructive feedback," says Borba. You could suggest, "Thank you for using your usual voice" or "My ears enjoy your voice." That worked well for my daughter. Any time she requested something respectfully, I accepted it and thanked her.

Refuse to let it annoy you. Find a peaceful moment and reassure your kid that there's a rule change: if he whines, you 're not going to respond. "From now on, if he whines, hold the face expression totally blank," advises Borba. Answer the kid politely that you can't hear what he needs while he whines, so you're going to react while he's talking with a pleasant voice.

Be sure the kid knows what "talking politely" entails. Maybe she doesn't really recognize she's whining — or maybe she doesn't even grasp what the term implies. The easiest way to clarify it is to capture both her whiny and sweet voices and then hand them back to her. (Make it obvious that you're using the recording to help her think, not to make her feel terrible.) They have a script to replicate when you tell them.

Hang in there. "Some parents claim, 'I attempted it yesterday, and it didn't work,'" Borba says. "But consider modifying one of your own habits: it will not happen immediately." I saw a difference in Elizabeth after a month.

Sadly, if you don't help your child learn good coping methods, the moaning can grow worse and influence his potential interactions. "Nobody wants to be around a whiny baby," says Borba. "bear in mind that your aim is to help your baby be the best he can be — and the time it takes is worth it."

2.9 Guide To Toddler Napping

To help their development and progress, Toddlers have to nap. Their minds and bodies are through at very high levels, and they require time to refresh and digest all the new things that they know for the time.

Furthermore, kids are little humans, much like adults, who are agitated without adequate sleep. The kid would be much satisfied and perform healthier with enough sleep, which would also reduce the intensity of the outbursts (but we can't promise to absolutely cut them out!).

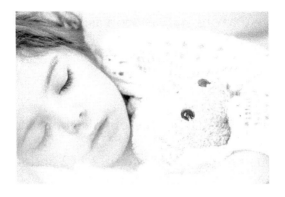

When babies reduce naps to one?

On average, the change of babies from two naps to one nap is around 15-18 months old. Many 13-14-month-olds continue the process slowly, but moving too early will lead to a major mess with staying up at night, waking up too early in the morning, or taking really short naps.

Bear in mind that your kid will now have to remain alert for 5 hours prior to nap AND after the nap during the shift to one nap. To several younger kids, that is no small accomplishment. They will be able to handle it for one day without breaking down or displaying any indicators of being too drained, just not quite every day.

How many naps will my little baby take?

Some kids can have two naps, on average, until they are 15-18 months old, and only then have one nap until they reach 3-4 years old. Nonetheless, nap changes can differ quite a little.

Some babies move to one nap as soon as 12 months old, while certain 5-year-olds are also napping at times.

How do children stop napping?

The typical age when kids quit napping is about the ages of 3 and 4, with some falling at the age of 2 1/2 and some falling only before age 5 and above.

There are usually 3 indicators that the child will be done napping, including:

1. Unable to fall asleep early enough to get ample awake time until bedtime.

2. Staying up at bedtime very late and sleeping fewer than 9-10 hours at night.

3. Miss the nap four or more days a week, no matter how quickly or late you 're giving it.

Of course, if your kid loses the nap, he may require one to two days a week while he gets accustomed to the new routine. This will take many weeks to a few months for the child to lose this long-term every day.

How long will a baby's naps be?

When an infant has been moving to 2 naps after 9 months of age, both naps will be at least one hour long to be deemed recover. Right before the switch to one nap, we often see 4 hours of awake time between both cycles of sleep and 10 1/2 hours of overall night-time sleep falls.

Often, before the move to one nap, one nap is a shorter catnap of 30-45 minutes, too, though not often. Typically speaking, if all naps are longer than an hour and your kid is over 13 months old, you may want to start moving into one nap.

When the baby starts doing only one nap, the sleep usually lasts 2-3 hours, before they are at least two years old. The nap will range from 1-3 hours after two years, based on the age and how much sleep it receives at night. Many babies require fast, restorative naps, and others require prolonged nights to feel rested, but the average will stay fairly consistent over a 24-hour span.

Quick naps are a growing parental concern, and you're not alone! First, evaluate if age-appropriate is the "short nap" for your kid. For example, a 17-month-old who still takes two naps may take one or two shorter naps because it's time to switch to a single nap. Or, a 3-year-old can require just a 45-60 minute nap a day at the end of the napping to get to bedtime. There is a distinction between having a brief nap and not getting adequate rest compared with getting the sleep that she wants.

If your kid will sleep longer and isn't, there are a number of factors your kid cannot sleep long enough:

• Pacifier – If you started using a pacifier lately, the child

might have difficulty changing it. If it was less than 2-3 weeks, then you might just want to give her more time. You will need to do some sleep training if it's been longer, give her a new lovey, or try offering the pacifier back before she's able to quit the nap for good.

• Sleep Associations – When you are not having your kid fall asleep at the start of his nap, he or she might not be able to return back to sleep without your assistance. Still, now that he is bigger, he's up already! Studying him how to fall asleep at nap time on his own could help to lengthen the naps.

• Timetable – occasionally, naps become short due to the wrong routine. Your infant may be under- or over-tired, or at night he/she might sleep "too long" based on the amount of sleep he or she may take in general.

• Hunger – Did you make sure that the next meal for your baby doesn't land in the midst of a nap? If so, beef the food or meal before the nap.

The nap may be short for other reasons, but these are the main culprits.

My kid won't nap without me.

When your kid doesn't sleep outside of your chest, neck, or with you in bed, so that is a sleep relationship. Unless you find it to be, this is not a "problem." When you have the time to sleep with your kid every day, and you love it, so perfect! Enjoy it now, or the sleep WILL go soon!

Nevertheless, if you love napping with your baby but have certain stuff to do, such as cleaning the home, preparing dinner, or caring for his sister, then it might not be feasible for you to take a 2-3 hour nap per day or keep your baby on your lap. If that's the case, so with some subtle sleep encouragement, you 'd definitely want to focus on helping your kid know how to sleep more peacefully.

My kids naps too long

First, a nap is usually not "too long" unless it in the middle of the night causes insomnia, or you have another medical concern. If your "problem" is that bedtime gets too late or your kid wakes too early for the day, then this is more of a scheduling problem. Cutting the nap and/or shifting the schedule can address that.

Should I give my baby lunch before or after the nap?

Some people offer lunch before the nap, so if your kid is anything like mine, we had "Lunch # 1" before the nap and "Lunch # 2" after the nap. For all, at 11:00 a.m., the kid could have lunch, and dinner is not before 6:00 p.m. or so. That's 7 hours, and a number of kids would have to eat a lot of "snacks" to dine. Do yourself a favor and literally attach it to another "lunch." What it's called is not even relevant!

2.10 Toddlers Don't Share Stuff

this phase of social and cognitive development is when children acquire "an awareness of themselves and others as independent persons." While based on language learning, this stage becomes most intense about two and starts to drop off around age three. "Children begin to recognize themselves as a human-they have common and specific traits, both physical and emotional, from others. This sets up disputes to some extent, "Moore says. "Children have clear expectations and interests — part of this is their possession over items. I am me. That's mine. It is an absolutely natural stage that we want to see kids going through.

Wendy Burch Jones, a mom of two from Scarborough, Ont., is in the throes of this with Zachary, a two-year-old. "He's got an older brother, and he found out early," she notes. Burch Jones has taught grade one and is used to diffuse disputes over exchanging, but she says that her expertise in the classroom is not comparable with the home scene. "We wrestled over a motor car this morning. We have 100, yet each chose the black one. "Most of the time, Burch Jones, encourages her boys to work everything out themselves — which psychologists suggest is the safest approach for parents — but she will intervene when squabbles transform into crying when things get hard. "We are going back to taking turns. I tell them how to inquire politely instead of their go-to move, which is catching.

Moore convinces parents that this is a healthy stage of life for infants, and you shouldn't feel the need to limit it. "The creation of freedom and autonomy is essential to children," he says. "If two kids play with toys and keep saying 'mine,' teach them to understand that the other kid also has feelings and an interest in that toy — we call it 'perspective taking.'"

Sharing notions can be learned early on. "Even babies will show cooperation with adults," Moore notes. But, until fairly late, certain aspects - such as fairness - will not be understood. He offers an example: "When you offer a three-year-old the option of keeping two treats for himself or trading one with someone else, he is more inclined to take two for himself — but he may share on occasion, he is more inclined to share them with friends than with strangers."

The identification of what is theirs (and what is not) is a characteristic that never entirely vanishes. We're still involved in what's ours, Moore says, but luckily it's not articulated as strongly later as it is during this early childhood period. "The notion of autonomy was established sometime later."

Burch Jones considers the advantages of the neediness of her sons. "It's fascinating to follow Zach stand out as a unique individual, and attempt to manage and test his world," she says. "The flip side of the whiny 'mine' stage is that he ends up playing together with his older brother. Watching their relationship develop, and watching their personalities unfold, was magical.

2.11 Potty Training

Toilet training is a big move forward for babies — and their guardians. The mystery to attaining greatness? Patience and timing.

It's time?

The success of potty training depends on physical, developmental, and cognitive achievements, not age. Most kids are displaying signals that they are eager for toilet training around 18 - 24 months. Some might not be able until they're three years old, however. There's no hurry in there. If you begin too soon, your kid might need to be trained for longer.

Is your baby ready? Ask yourself:

• Would your kid walk to the bathroom and sit on the toilet?

• Can your child pull pants down and pull them back again?

• Is your child able to stay dry for up to 2 hours?

• Can your kid follow simple directions, and obey them?

• Is your child willing to express where he needs to go?

• Does your kid appear focused on wearing the "big-kid" underwear or the toilet?

If you replied mainly yes, maybe your kid's ability, if you responded mostly no, you may want to sit tight — especially if your kid is about to face a significant change, like a move or a new sibling's entry.

There's key in your preparation. Let your kid's motivation guide the process instead of your Potty training eagerness. Try not to match the achievement or difficulty of potty training with the intellectual ability or obstinacy of your child. Also, note that mistakes are possible, so deterrence should not play a role in the formation. Plan potty training when, for a few months, you or a caretaker can devote time and effort to being consistent every day.

Ok, hold on, go!

When the time is right to start potty training:

• Pick your terms. Consider which phrases to use for body fluids in your kid. Don't use offensive phrases, like gross or stinky terms.

• Making equipment ready. Place a toilet in your toilet or, at first, wherever your kid spends much of his or her day. Ask your child to continue sitting on the potty toilet dressed. Making sure the feet of your child are on the concrete or a chair. To talk about the toilet, using the simple, appropriate terms. To show their purpose, you may dump the contents of a used diaper into the potty chair and the toilet. Let your kid empty the toilet.

• Potty breaks are planned. Have your child rest on the potty chair or toilet at two-hour time frames without a diaper for a few mins, including first thing every morning and right after the naps. For boys, it is always better to practice sitting urination and then switch to standing up after finishing stool training. Remain with your kid and read a book or play with a gadget while he or she is sitting. Have your child stand up anytime he or she needs to. Even if your child is just sitting there, bid admiration for attempting — and reassure your kid that he or she may try again later. When you're away from home with your kids, carry the potty chair along with you.

• Have a go-easy! React quickly when you notice any signs that your child may require using the bathroom — such as squirming, kneeling, or holding the genital region— Help your child get to know these cues, stop whatever he or she is doing, and head out to the toilet. Admire your kid to remind you when to move. Put your kids in garments that are loose and easy to remove.

• Explain about hygiene. Tell women to spread their legs and carefully wipe away from front to back to stop the vagina or bladder from bringing bacteria from the rectum. Afterward, ensure that the kid washes his or her hands.

• stop using the diapers. Your child may be big enough to trade diapers for training pants or undergarments after a few weeks of effective potty breaks and remaining dry over the day. Feast on the transformation. If he or she can't keep dry, let your kid revert to diapers. For constructive motivation, try utilizing a badge or star map.

Take a break if your kid avoids using the bathroom or toilet, or doesn't get the feel of it after a few days. Odds are he or she is still not ready. Trying to push your child when he or she is not ready can contribute to a stressful struggle for control. Seek again in a month or two.

Training in the Night

Usually, it takes longer to achieve nap time and especially at night training. Most kids between the ages of 5 and 7 may stay dry in the evening. Meanwhile, when your child sleeps, use reusable training pants and bed-covers.

Accidents also arise

Dealing with accidents:

• Remain calm. Don't criticize, chastise, or disgrace your kid. You might say, "This time you missed. Sooner, you'll get to the toilet the next time."

• Prepare. Keep an underpants and garments change handy, especially in school or child care.

When to support

If your child appears prepared for potty training but has trouble, talk to your doctor. He or she can give you advice and check if there is an underlying issue.

Chapter 3: Preschoolers (3 to 5 years)

Way to discipline a preschooler needs a blend of science and art. It needs some significant strength, too. What operated last week might not be effective anymore.

Patience and persistence with the 3-, 4-, or 5-year-old will be crucial to solving behavioral issues. Around the same time, you would need to occasionally make use of a little trial and error to see what learning methods would fit better for your family.

3.1 Typical Actions of A Preschooler

The development of a preschooler means your kid would want to be autonomous. This search for individuality will bring new behavioral and discipline-related barriers to parenting. And, your child may enjoy playing with different behaviors to see exactly how you're going to react.

The transition to pre-school may cause anxiety about separation in your child.

Or, he can have anxieties regarding communicating with other teachers and babies.

Children might still be playing with breaking norms and

limitations at this age and can demonstrate defiance. They may feel frustrated that they cannot do what they want to do because their motor skills are not yet as refined as they are. Even these stresses and anxieties will contribute to issues with actions such as aggression, talking back, dawdling, and more.

Preschoolers have a fundamental sense of what is right from wrong. They should obey basic guidelines, and most approach adults to satisfy them. They do not, however, follow the logic of adults, so they occasionally fail to make healthy decisions.

Even though they can learn stronger self - control, your child still requires a lot of research in this field. They may shout, say mean things, or display outbursts. They also challenge laws and restrictions but will continue to gain a deeper sense of the actual results of their actions.

Common Difficulties

Telling lies is a key problem in preschoolers. Sometimes their tales are an effort to get out of the difficult situation, and sometimes they just use their imagination and creativity to tell stories that are far-fetched.

Whining is yet another common problem in pre-school years. Preschoolers often think that, if you first say no, begging and complaining will compel you to change your mind. But remember, once they succeed in irritating you once into compliance, they will be sure they will be able to do it again.

Baby speaking is close to the top of the list of irritating pre-school behaviors in many homes. But it can be a regular part of pre-school growth to return to baby talk. Preschoolers often do this to gain publicity. Other times, because of stress or anxiety, they regress. For instance, a child may start using baby talk right before entering kindergarten because he's anxious about the transformation.

While preschoolers always want to be supportive, they want to demonstrate their freedom as well. They're commonly told, "No! "In telling them to do something just to observe how you're going to react.

Many preschoolers have acquired a degree of dominance over-emotional outbursts but have also not developed adequate self-regulation to avoid occasional violent behavior. Hitting, punching and biting may also be a problem.

Strategies for Discipline That Work

A successful punishment will include harsh outcomes that discourage repetitive misbehavior and beneficial results that inspire your child to continue doing the good work. Although the strategy will be adapted to the personality of the infant, the following disciplinary methods are typically more appropriate with preschoolers.

Glory be to decent behavior

Provide much support and recognition for promoting good conduct. Only see to it that the support is real. Instead of saying, "You are the world's best boy," say, "thanks for bringing your dish in the sink when I told you to."

Place your child in time - out.

Using an immediate time-out for significant breaches of the law, such as violence. And, using it for those moments that your child doesn't follow a message like, "If you're not cleaning up the toys right now, then you're going to have to go out on time." Younger preschoolers will require a time-out space, although most 5-year-olds may handle doing time-out in a seat or other quiet place.

Throw Privileges Away

If the preschooler fails to head out on schedule, even if the crime is not worth a couple of minutes away from the game, seek to revoke certain rights. Rip away the perks of a beloved car, game, or TV for the rest of the day.

Creating a System of Rewards

If your child deals with a certain trait, including spending all night in their own room, build a sticker map. Then inform them that if they win any stickers (say three or five), they will get a bigger prize, say picking up a fun video to watch. Reward programs should be phased out gradually until the child has mastered the skills it requires to achieve its objectives.

3.2 Attempting To Prevent Future Problems

Risk reduction can be the best approach when it comes to punishing a preschooler. Stay on top by bearing in mind circumstances that your child will likely find difficult.

Many preschoolers fail whether they are starving, overtired, or exhausted to control their impulses. So pack snacks, allow plenty of rest, and schedule trips for when your child will probably be at its best.

Create a daily routine so that your child knows all day long what is anticipated of them. Preschoolers perform their work because there is a ton of structure.

Creating simple guidelines and boundaries, too. Explain the goals when you reach unfamiliar scenarios (such as how to conduct in the library), and alert the child about the repercussions about violating the law.

Many of the behavioral issues experienced by preschoolers are the product of their inability to control their emotions — especially anger. Teach basic conflict control techniques for your preschooler. Blow bubbles with your kids, for example, as a means of encouraging them to take slow, soothing breaths and encourage them to use "bubble breaths" when they get crazy.

Set guidelines around offensive conduct in the building. Teach your child that feeling angry is okay but not okay to offend anybody or destroy property.

Mistakes Parents Make With Preschoolers

Often, the preschooler can appear to have the inherent power to drive you beyond the very limits of endurance, even on a productive day.

Don't be scared, mums, and fathers. You are not isolated in this. Pregnant schoolchildren desire their freshly discovered freedom. Yet they like their carers' deep attention and affection too.

Michele Borba, EdD, author of The Major Book of Parenting Strategies, states, "These ages (3-5) are perhaps the most parenting involved and stressful.

Here are eight typical errors pre-school parents make and a few clever solutions to either prevent or overcome problems.

1. So many straying from habits

Consistency is essential for preschoolers, says child psychologist Tanya Remer Altmann, writer of Mommy Calls: Dr. Tanya Addresses the Top 101 Infant and Toddlers Questions from Parents.

When you're not aligned with your schedule, preschoolers get puzzled and may act more or toss more temper tantrums. Altmann says, "If you let them do something sometimes, and sometimes you don't, they don't understand."

Your kid possibly needs to ask why Mommy let her play on the field for 10 minutes last time when school came out, but this time she needs her to get into the car right away. Or why did Mommy sit down with her last night for 10 minutes when she fell asleep, but now she insists she can't.

Repair it: Be consistent around the board — whether training, sleeping patterns or mealtime schedules are concerned.

Altmann states that if the schedule is 90 percent of the time successful and the child is doing good, then you are, so a

small exception may be Fine.

2. Pessimistic Focus

It's easy to hone in on the negative actions of your child — like screaming and shouting — and ignore the good ones.

Altmann believes parents want to rely on what their preschoolers don't want to do. "They'll be telling, 'Don't strike. Don't fire at them. Don't say pants poopy, "she notes.

Fix it: Note whether your kid does a successful thing and praise good behavior.

The incentive for good behavior can be your congratulations, or it may be offering your kid a huge embrace or kiss. "For preschoolers, these sorts of stuff often go a long way," says Altmann.

Say to your boy, "I like the fact you sat and listened silently," or "It was nice when you were so sweet to the kid on the playground."

3. Missing Alarm Signals

If parents are in the throes of a temper tantrum, they sometimes attempt to negotiate with them, chanting, "Calm down, calm down." Yet that's like attempting to communicate with a goldfish, Borba says. "When you can still distract or anticipate, you have power immediately beforehand, but once the tantrum is in full force, you've lost it. The kid doesn't hear you."

Fix it: Work it out and know what the usual warning signals for your child are, says Borba. The common ones are hunger, tiredness, and boredom.

So don't carry your kid to the store until she's napped or you've stashed in your bag a nutritious snack.

4. Encouraging Whining

Would you moaning about your kid make you crazy? For e.g., does it push you up the wall when your child begins weeping right before dinner while cooking food, "I want to go to the park," or "I want to go to play with Riley."

Borba tells parents often consider giving in to these whines, but this only strengthens the attentive behavior. Your child's going to find out which buttons to press and then move them away.

"This is the era of getting the kids out of their shells," she notes. "Watch out, because they are working out what works."

Put it right: Forget.

You're best prepared with action that isn't hostile, like a moan or sulk, if you don't react to it at all. When you are persistent, says Borba, your child's likely to figure, "Oh, that didn't work."

5. Over-scheduling the kid

Families also set up a variety of events, such as dance lessons and music courses. Then they wonder why their kid doesn't get into bed and fall asleep immediately after so many tasks that had to make her tired.

The question, says Altmann, is they're all wound up, and they need time to cool down. Each child requires time off, and she says, particularly preschoolers. This can be quite stressful when the child is in a nursery for two hours or there all day.

Fix it: Don't overwork or move the kid from one operation to another. Offer your child room when he comes home from school to unwind with free play.

6. Underestimating play Value

Many parents believe that to give them an advantage, and they will sign up their kids for enrichment programs. Yet this still is not the case.

What is most enriching at this age is free to play, explains dr. Lawrence J. Cohen, writer of Playful Parenting. That includes (make-believe) dramatic play, roughhousing, and larking around.

"Fair play is the best to grow children's minds," he notes. "Naturally, kids will give themselves the right amount of challenge in play — not too easy or too hard."

Fix it: Give free playtime and room to your boy. Recall that preschoolers describe playing as "what you do when you know what to do."

Free option — the voluntary side of play — is significant, says Cohen. "Preschoolers tend to clean or do housework because it's playing. It's not on their job list. They've decided to do something because they're only doing it for pleasure," he states.

7. Distraction by the daily routine

The child may play well alone, but that doesn't imply that he or she won't be searching for attention. "When parents don't sit on the floor and play with them, there is something kids lose out on," Cohen notes.

Not only are parents not sitting down and playing, but also parents become disturbed too quickly by their mobile phone, email, or other multitasking. "Kids aren't dumb," says Cohen. "We ask whether we are paying good attention or not."

Adjust it: Set a timer, be positive, and keep active with your child during your allocated play date.

"A half-hour of focused play when you're offering your full attention and don't care about dinner or jobs," Cohen notes, "is better than the entire day where you're just half paying attention."

8. Responding to Lies

Cohen claims lying really freaks out people. He encourages parents to see the actions as more experimentation than "a spiritual matter."

"It's a major cognitive development when the children decide to deceive," he says. "It's sort of thrilling and a little frightening. It's got an emotional impact, but then parents stress out and have hallucinations of their kid in prison, and they feel really nervous and worried."

Correct it: Don't overreact. Know that telling a lie or two is a natural part of raising your kids.

So don't hang yourself up on the fib, Cohen notes. For starters, if your little Pinocchio insists that he has anything to do with a spill, you might honestly reply, "You're feeling terrible about that, and I understand."

3.3 Bedtime Battles

With newly discovered freedom, young children may be a hassle to relax in the nighttime. All that momentum will either escalate through pre-school bedtime fights or become a quiet road to sleep.

Start With A Consistent Routine

And if your preschooler has never had a consistent bedtime routine, there's no time like the moment to initiate one. This will take your child a few days to get adjusted to a new schedule to adapt. Your child will adjust really easily, and will soon be looking forward to the new routine.

If one night you overlook or attempt to miss a move, you'll definitely hear about it! That's because daily rituals provide young children with a sense of calm, continuity, and health. If a kid thinks he can foresee what's happening — even though he's throwing up a fight about it — he seems a little bit more in charge of the life. Through them, it's the reverse of the disorder.

Having a fixed schedule in Bedtime would often give you the stability you need when you're tired. You will love a map at the end of a busy day — either a visual document or one hung on your wall — that shows you what the next move is! You'll soon even be able to use the schedule as a gentle reference away from NOT everything on the board.

"Sweetie, I'd love to show all of your drawings in superblocks, but we can't do it right now. Let's look at the map and see what's next. We will look at those amazing inventions when you wake up in the morning!"

Characteristics of a healthy bedtime routine

Firstly talk of the basics:

• Pjs

• Cleaning teeth

• A bathroom stop

• Warmth (snuggles and hugs for Bedtime);

• Tucking into bunk

• Turn the lights off.

Then back up from there to connect to the items that matter to you and to your kids. Do you want to have a toy pickup time? This is a fantastic habit of learning for your child. Yet maybe it blends in with the bedtime schedule or not.

Is there a bedtime snack you can place on the chart? This will support a kid who has a propensity to climb into bed and announce that he is "hungry." Nothing can ruin a nice sleep in a bed like a crying, hungry boy. If they've had a nutritious snack and some drink, so you realize their hunger or thirst announcement is just a stalling strategy or something they only need to cope with before breakfast comes around. Just having a little bedtime snack makes it easier to say, "No, you've had your snack, and now it's time to settle down in bed."

Shower or no shower?

To some kids, bath time isn't a relaxing experience because they're scared of water, or they play in the bathtub too joyfully. Yet, for others, it is a classic feature of a restful bedtime ritual. If your child doesn't succeed with it, don't stress. Find a perfect way and incorporate it into your days.

Liquids and Bedtime

Whether your kid tends to wet the bed, always has a leaky pad, or gets up in the middle of the night to go potty, it's a smart idea to avoid all kinds of liquids after dinner time. So that means hydrating them throughout the day is very necessary.

You will then probably get one tiny cup of water in the toilet at Bedtime. We are done partying for the night until it is clean.

Speed Down To Rest

It's necessary to help your child wind down from daylight. Shut off or switching off all the child's technological gadgets an hour before Bedtime. It will sound like a challenging concept to obey, but if you do, you can see a change in the willingness of your child to settle down for bed. For every bedtime woe, it isn't a cure-all, but it's definitely an important component supported up by good science.

Several experiments have found that TVs, computers, and even our tiny mobile gadgets produce enough light to distort the brain and facilitate wakefulness. They may throw away our circadian rhythms sufficiently to interrupt sleep cycles, especially in kids.

This is enticing to conceive about children's toys as a help in our parenting. Yet they may be a hindrance to the bedtime ambitions until dinner time. Power down so you can get to sleep on time.

The Human Touch

Nearly every kid likes to cuddle and be close to Bedtime. I hope you will create some of the better memories from parenting at this time of your day. Choose a place for them to move from cuddling to bed quickly. It could be on your pillow or a neighboring sofa. If you've reached a nice spot, stay with it. The continuity lets you preserve your schedule. So make sure you snuggle, kiss, cuddle, and let your kid hear the expressions of affection and assertiveness.

Learn aloud and recall.

In other cultures, Bedtime is a synonym in reading books. Let your child pick one or two favorite books (not the longest) and read them aloud in a gentle voice. Escape the frightening afternoon tales and dramatic sounds! Children gain too much in childhood by repetition. Children are often oriented towards learning the same tales children enjoy the most, as they understand more and reinforce the ideas in their heads with increasing hearing. I consider sticking through the book at Bedtime, which appears to them the most soothing, even though you sound like a robot doing the same stuff over and over.

When the kids reach high school age, you can pick a longer chapter book each night and read a chapter or section of a chapter. At that point, your kids may start looking forward to Bedtime in a different way, because they want to know what's next.

If this reading period takes on a life of its own — too lengthy for Bedtime or too much suspense — you may want to switch it into the living room early in the evening and reduce the bedtime routine afterward.

Make a final stop in the pit.

Taking a minute for the last toilet break and a quick drink of tea if you want to read to your kid before bed. You would just have to use your parental experience at that stage to decide whether your kid just wants to go potty again or is searching for a reason to get out of bed.

Slip into a warm space

Eventually, you're placing your kid inside their bunk. Make sure the sheets are tightly tucked in, the covers match the temperature, the space is dark enough, and the closets are locked — believe me on this one! Apart from this, the cleaner and neater space are, the easier to get their minds relaxed at night. Admittedly, for several years, some kids won't know for neatness, but others do know and will not be able to verbalize their choice at a young age.

Tell 1-3 stuff good about your day. Research even suggests it is a healthy idea to finish the day on a productive note!

Send hugs and kisses, even sing a song and tell goodnight. Starting and finishing your child's day provides a healthy and stable atmosphere for them. Let each parent say goodnight, if at all necessary, even though one parent shoulder more daily load.

Sample Plan

• Cookies at Bedtime

• Pick up toys

• Take shower

• Wear pajamas

• Clean teeth

• Cuddle

• Read a story

• Bathroom stop

• move into bed

Be sure all the tougher things occur before the relaxing and snuggling and singing incentive! When they appear to get confused, this will help you keep them online.

Shuffling the Sleep Lady

You can revisit The Shuffle if you adhere to a new sleep

schedule for a few weeks, and your child is having difficulty going to sleep. Beware about not staying too long in one location by traveling every three days.

Use a Chart for Sleep Manners

When your kid is fond of stamps and stickers, try creating a list of sleep etiquette. You can do it quickly, and have your child interested. Pick from 3 to 4 forms to sleep and describe them respectfully, such as "lay in your own bed all night."

At Bedtime, draw focus and think about the chart of your infant, particularly though it appears they are "tuning out." Be specific on the habits you want to see more of. In the morning, apart from the stickers or tags, make sure you provide plenty of kisses and appreciation.

The purpose of the sleep behavior chart is to set goals and evaluate your and your child's behavior in improving or modifying it. I know that stickers and stars will not be motivational enough to improve the behavior of a boy, but having the poster as a reminder is a nice way to inform them about how Bedtime looks like.

Carry on with it

My best advice to you is to stick to the routine that you are developing. Tweak things the way you like to, and stretch as life demands, so don't give it up because it feels painful. For them, it's necessary to end the day well for your pre-schooler and how they sleep at night. You make them calm down and go into restful, deep sleep quicker than they will without the ease of a schedule.

3.4 Stop Wetting The Bed

You 're irritated. You are full of fatigue. Your kid is still in kindergarten-and at night; they still wet the bed. After dinner, you have probably been reducing the liquids. In the middle of the night, you have woken up your kids and asked them to go to the bathroom. Yet no luck.

You 're not alone on that. Families frequently panic about bedwetting in their kids, an issue described as "unintentional urination in kids 5 years of age or older." Yet, in fact, only 15 percent of U.S. kids actually wet the bed at age 5.

I referred to Charles Kwon, MD, a clinical nephrologist, and Audrey Rhee, MD, a child urologist to support parents overcome this problem.

Should I worry?

Dr. Kwon claims bedwetting bed isn't a problem unless the kid is 7.

You will want to speak to your child's primary care provider or a clinical nephrologist or urologist if your kid is older than 7 and always wetting the toilet. The actual problem is usually a not yet grown bladder.

Also, remember that about 15 percent of children 5 years of age or older actually stop wetting the bed every year.

"If I come across a child wetting the bed, it's significantly more likely to be a boy. He usually has no such medical problems, "states Dr. Kwon.

Dr. Kwon says parents are typically frustrated because it's a constant problem-so everybody wants some sleep. There are also concerns that there's a bedwetting family background as well. Doctors suggest: To prevent bedwetting

• Nights change to beer. Increase the intake of fluid earlier in the day and reduce it later in the day.

• Timing of breaks in the shower. Get your kid on a frequent urination schedule and right before bedtime (every two to three hours).

• Be positive. Help your kid feel better about progress by making successes continuously rewarded.

• Eliminate irritants to the bladder. Start by removing caffeine

at night (such as chocolate milk and cacao). And if that doesn't work, cut citrus juices, flavor enhancers, dyes (particularly red) and sweeteners. Most parents don't know that any of these will irritate the bladder of a boy.

• Stop thirst overloading. Offer your child a bottle of water, if schools approve, and they can drink regularly all day. After training, that prevents excessive thirst.

• Focus on how constipation can be a cause. Since the rectum is just behind the bladder, constipation problems may pose themselves, particularly at night, as a concern for the bladder. It affects around one-third of kids wetting the bed, while kids are unlikely to recognize or disclose constipation details.

• Don't wake the kids up for urination. Waking up a child spontaneously at night and telling them to urinate on command is not the solution, either. It would offer even more sleeplessness and anger.

• Later sojourn. Kids are also heavy sleepers, but they often don't get enough sleep.

• Cut the screen time back, particularly around bedtime. Improving sleep hygiene can help slow down their minds, so they can sleep better.

• Should not resort to penalty. It doesn't make them improve to get mad at your kids. Should not include confrontation in the process.

Medications: not usually recommended

However, there are medications (including a synthetic version of a hormone) that can treat bedwetting. I will not recommend them until another doctor has already placed an infant on the drug.

."Side effects do happen. And it's a partial patch, a band-aid cure when the final answer is what we want."

Does my child want to improve?

Families also question if a kid is deliberately bedwetting. Parents are likely to say, "Do they not want to do any better? "Dr. Kwon also assures parents that this is not usually their responsibility, nor is it the responsibility of their infant. "I advise them not to get too worried, as it always addresses this problem on its own," he says.

Dr. Rhee says that communicating with your child is always necessary to see whether there is some incentive for improvement. If they are inspired to improve, the answer may be a bedwetting warning.

You may either add the alarm to the underwear of the infant or place it on the bedside table. When the moisture is sensed by the system, the alarm goes off. Yet if the infant is not driven individually, the warning will have little value for the infant, and could only frustrate the family more.

"If they are still drinking alcohol late at night and eating what they shouldn't consume, then investing in an expensive bedwetting system doesn't make sense. So, I question a child specifically if bedwetting disturbed them, to figure out whether it was the disappointment of the parents that took the child to the appointment or on their own, "says Dr. Rhee.

When the child becomes older and has chances to go to overnight parties and weekend excursions, bedwetting will impact their confidence and social life. It is more likely to inspire the kid to fix the dilemma and prevent embarrassment.

When bedwetting means more serious problems

Bed-wetting is rarely a precursor of something more critical, including:

• Sleep apnea – Dr. Rhee will examine more whether an infant snores a lot or displays symptoms of sleep apnea. Otherwise, this is not the first screening test for an infant with bedwetting issues.

• Urinary tract infections (UTIs) – A measurement of urine will diagnose such diseases, which is a standard check physician would prescribe anytime bedwetting is a problem.

• Diabetes – Diabetes can also be detected in children by urine sample.

Age is important to remember whether a kid still has daytime incontinence. Kids will generally outgrow the issue. "Around 20 percent of children in the nursery had daytime incontinence. Yet only 5 percent of teenagers have such signs, "notes Dr. Kwon.

3.5 The Picky Eater

If only it was as easy as looking into our old Magic 8 Balls ® to find out if it's "very doubtful" or "decidedly so," it would be the correct thing to do for our children to refuse to stop at the Good Humor ® truck on the way home from school. Such worries, along with the problem of raising children in a fast-food, advertising-filled nation, are causing us to raise children whose diets are primarily pasta and chicken nuggets. The truth is that when they become teens and adults, we don't know if regulating food choices for our children will lead to food problems. But we can be certain that their growing

bodies are not good at relying entirely on processed food.

Here are some of the causes people end up with kids that do not consume well:

1. Parents are frightened to say no. It's not enough because they don't want to make a binger of ice cream. It's also that serving our kids is a way to foster and express our respect for them. Giving them treats such as french toast or chocolate chip cookies is so enticing just to see their happy faces, particularly if this was one of the ways our parents expressed their affection. The problem is, will we split this loop with nutritious foods, and show our love?

2. Parents think that eating processed food in moderation is ok for kids. Even if parents do not indulge themselves, it's suggested that children may consume it "in balance," so what precisely is "moderation?" Once per week, then? Twice a day? What will be a normal level of a substance like fake color, related to hyperactivity by several studies? Perhaps we're lulled into believing that kids require years to go before they begin to care about calories or fat. Yet the fact is that even infants have the early signs of plaque in their lungs, adolescent obesity is called an epidemic, and Type 2 diabetes is also way too prevalent in youngsters, previously just an adult illness.

3. Suggested by physicians and provided by schools. Most of our pediatricians advise us why we will give our children Cheerios ® beginning at the age of 10 months so that they can focus on their pincer grip, never knowing that the cereals are heavily refined and full of basic carbohydrates that easily transform into sugar in the body. However, everyone with children understands that they fine-tune their pincer grip by picking up the tiniest specks of soil from the floor and placing them in their mouth skillfully. The other shocking where kids get introduced to nutritious food is the hospital, in addition to the doctor's office. It starts with the mama and me classes, where kids are served goldfish crackers to snack on, despite being rich in salt and basic graham crackers, or, worse, carbohydrates which are little different than cookies hidden in a package labeled "crackers," next to apple juice, another large sugar serving. By preschool, my children were provided brownies or cupcakes, sometimes with bright pink or blue icing, to celebrate a birthday or vacation at least once a week.

4. Creating a pre-packaged meal is alluringly simple because we realize our kids are going to feed. "Nuking" chicken nuggets, which have been medically designed to satisfy the

little ones or to cook pasta, require far less time to produce a dinner than waiting in the kitchen for a couple of hours. Understandably, after working the whole day inside or outside the home, that might not be so alluring, particularly in our excessively-scheduled, extremely intense culture, where spending hours working in the kitchen is no longer called time well spent.

Whatever the reason, the problem is, what do you do now? If you have a blank start for a newborn or with an older kid seeking to shift paths, here are few ideas.

1. Make sure the kids are genuinely hungry for dinner (or whatever food you serve). So don't let them eat any candy or too much bread after school, for example. Whether it is two to three hours until mealtime, just have fruits and veggies, whether hungry.

2. Only have the food that you would like them to consume in your house. "Sorry, we don't have any Oreos" is way easier than, "Sorry, there are no Oreos you can get."

3. Let them play a part in any element of food preparation. My son once discovered some online recipes that were child-friendly and was completely excited about creating and consuming ants-on-a-log (nut butter and celery raisins). Or, let

them cut or slice any vegetables or even switching on the blender with your close supervision. It just takes me half as long if my children help me make a dish, so it's worth it (usually!) because they're so much more involved in trying what they've made.

4. When you can lie down together and eat, do so. Children are often influenced by what their parents do, and they consume each other. Mind you, in the three years since we began eating with our kids, I have not had a relaxing dinner, but I feel hopeful that it will happen one day soon.

5. Don't pressure children into having food if they don't really want to. If my kid, the family's most picky eater, was younger and balked at the lentils and brown rice I had prepared for dinner, I would have provided simple, nutritious contingency choices that I knew she wanted, like a bunch of pistachio nuts or whole wheat tortillas and hummus. Eventually, whether she was dissatisfied with the replacement foods or excited to see others consume the lentils and beans, she started to eat it, too.

6. The child may have to try 10 to 15 times a new food before he's able to consume it. This is how it was with my daughter and vegetarian chili. She's enjoying it now, more or less

willingly, as long as I remove the broccoli and onions before I feed them!

7. Give the kids the same stuff that you eat. It is particularly beneficial when consuming solids is relatively new to your kids. As long so your kids can swallow the meal, there's no need why their home menu and restaurant menu should appear any different from yours. Through this way, they would have the chance to taste the flavors and colors of 'true' food and not become accustomed to the commonly provided fluffy, white food.

8. Your kids are wise! Interact with them. Explain why you want the improvements you 're making — that you value them and think for their teeth and bodies. You want them to grow up, and they feel safe as happy. They may not like the changes, but they should be helped to understand them.

9. Don't undervalue your children. My oldest was just getting his 8th birthday with 14 buddies, most of whom are consuming regular American fare. While he convinced me to serve daily pizza (I had refused for several birthdays), instead of chips, I placed out loads of grapes, sliced apples, and cucumbers all over the wall. Nearly all had gone by the party's end. I regarded that victory as mine!

Unpleasantly, we have no study yet that tells us more accurately than the Magic 8 Ball ® that refusing our kids junk food would hurt them, especially when they see their friends partaking in it. However, we do have a vast array of studies that show clearly how detrimental to health these artificial, fatty, sugar-processed foods are. Changing your kids' diet may sound overwhelming no matter how old they are, but as they grow older, it won't get easier, so now is the time to start! I think it may be possible.

This hasn't just worked for my family. For anyone else that I've seen practice these rules, this worked. You will do anything you want to raise safe and happy babies. Why Should you not offer attention to their diet too?

3.6 Recognize And Label Their Emotions

1. Offer young people a language for their thoughts. Use Moodz posters to help children recognize their thoughts and mark their feelings. Children may not have the vocabulary for what they mean but can understand the feeling on a child's face in the expression. Ask kids to point to the person that better reflects their own emotions on the poster and then show them the symbol for that emotion.

2. Use picture books as a resource to examine feelings - Pick books that explain the characters' facial expressions throughout the plot—select picture books with themes suitable for young, as well as adult, readers for older children. Read the book to children, observing the facial gestures, feelings, disagreements, behavior, and responses to the actors and results. Then, demonstrate the children the words for the feelings of the characters.

3. Play charades with emotions! - Write down a number of various feelings on paper slips and place them in a bag or cap. Let children take turns choosing an emotion to embody and carry out the feeling in front of the community, without saying. Then, the majority of the class will infer what emotion is being presented.

4. Tell them what it feels like. Recognizing the emotions of a person, and offering them a language for those thoughts, is very critical. For secondary children, this method is just as legitimate as for young children. Help children communicate how they feel, and thus behave, with tags for their feelings. For example, as children get upset if they don't get their way, suggest, "I can tell you 're feeling irritated right now." Stop using the term angry, or it's equivalents. Angry is being overstated. Teachers and parents may help young people

learn to properly mark their feelings themselves by marking their feelings for them.

5. Role-play involving kids – Use scenarios that exist in the school, let two kids at one-point role-play how they will behave in front of the class in a scenario. Let one kid behave like a bully, for example, when the other kid acts like the victim. For an example of role-playing, let all the kids think about how they would react if they found themselves in a specific circumstance.

6. Teach children to be mindful of their body language and the image it reflects. When children perform the part in a situation, encourage the viewer to examine the feelings and meanings the body language of the characters has conveyed. Most young people are entirely oblivious of what kind of meaning their body language is transmitting. By finding it out and marking the feelings it expresses, children may become more mindful and more in charge of their body language and understand more about the mechanism of identifying feelings.

7. Help children recognize that rage is a secondary feeling– They encounter another, sometimes overlooked, main emotion, such as disappointment, envy, shock, or humiliation before an individual feel angry. If a child says he's upset, help

him recognize and mark the primary emotion underlying the rage to grasp the feelings better and cope with it.

8. Show Empathy-Make them consider how the other individual thinks when they are engaged in a confrontation. Question them how they would behave if they had been in the shoes of the other. By teaching children to recognize and consider not just their own feelings but other people's feelings as well, teachers and parents may encourage young people to better mark and interpret emotions more effectively.

9. Help children link their feelings and body language – Ask children to remember a circumstance that made them feel good, unhappy, frustrated, or some other emotion. Let children draw a photo of facial expression to suit the emotion provided and then distribute the pictures among the community. Seeing the various images of children can help to decide how each kid sees each emotion.

10. To help children recognize their frustration more, encourage children to compose a brief story that explains a circumstance that caused them "angry" without utilizing the terms "hate," "angry," "evil," etc. This will enable children to recognize the emotions which trigger rage. Children may use the Moodz banner as a "Vocabulary list of emotions."

11. Help children appreciate various feelings by encouraging them to compose an acrostic piece in which each character of the name of emotion will reflect a cause to feel that way. For, e.g., the sentence "Give away my friend's secret" might start with G in guilt.

12. To help children recognize circumstances that lead them to encounter a particular emotion, encourage children to talk about the feelings they feel more often and what causes them to think that way. If children know that the same circumstance often causes them to feel unhappy or hurt, so they are likely to stop the problem or find a different way of coping with it. It should enable children to build effective strategies to cope with disagreements and feelings.

3.7 Anger Management Strategies

"Punch the cushions! "It's a growing piece of advice that kids get on how to cope with frustration. The premise behind this guide is that people either have to let out their frustration or erupt violently. There is sadly no scrap of proof that this is beneficial. In reality, rage after "venting" appears to repeat and escalate.

For starters, in one research, Brad Bushman annoyed student

participants at college by offering them assessments on an essay they had submitted, allegedly by another research participant. The incorrect evaluations were highly negative and contained remarks like "This is among the worst writings I've seen! "And very poor ratings on numerical qualities like organization, uniqueness, and clarity.

Then, participants either saw an image of their alleged critique and hit a punching bag while talking about that individual (venting situation), strike a punching bag while talking about exercising and physical activity (active coping condition), or simply sat down calmly for a few minutes (control condition). People in the state of venting subsequently recorded becoming angrier and behaving more violently as compared to the control group. The participants in the successful diversion community were less upset than the venting category but not less violent. Monitor community members, who had already been waiting, showed the lowest rates of rage and hostility.

Knowing the cycle of emotional control

So if hitting cushions is likely just to escalate the rage of kids, what better tactics should we offer our children? In order to address the issue, first, we need to step back to reflect on how feelings grow. This method model of emotion control describes five points at which users can adjust their emotional reactions:

1. Situation Management requires the quest for or avoidance of circumstances that are likely to cause specific emotions.

2. Condition Adjustment means doing something to alter a condition so that the mental effect improves.

3. Attentional Implementation involves utilizing diversion or dwelling on it to reduce or enhance emotional reactions.

4. Cognitive Change means adapting perspectives of an event that triggers emotions or judgments regarding an individual's ability to cope.

5. Response Manipulation means doing something after it has been developed to change the physiological, observational, or behavioral dimensions of an emotional response. Any manipulation strategy of the answer can help the dynamics, cycling back via earlier measures.

Parents should support kids in any step in the cycle of controlling emotions. Take the example of a kid being upset at a sibling for knocking over a tower block. Parents could influence situation selection by making sure the child is not tired or hungry and thus more prone to angrily respond.

Situation Adjustment may include predicting the mishap and instructing the child to shift the block tower to a position where knock-over is less possible. Attention Deployment may involve offering a snack or heading outdoors to divert the child from the tower that was tumbled. Cognitive progress may include demonstrating to the kid that the sibling unintentionally pushed it over, or that the tower can be quickly repaired in an even better way. Answer Modulation may include helping the child repair the structure, or urging the child to "use their language" to ask the sibling to step over or to help pick up the bricks.

Within this scheme, the first four steps reflect precedent-focused emotion regulation, since they govern processes involved in the processing of emotions. The final stage is responsive-focused management, because it involves adjusting what individuals are doing to cope with an anger that has already emerged in. Managing emotions early in the process rather than later is often easier and more effective.

Seen in this sense, it is not shocking that it is not sufficient to smash cushions to try and control the frustration. This does little to change the condition or the way it is perceived by youngsters.

How parents can teach the management of anger

Yeah, how do parents support kids' learn how to handle their emotions? Below are a few support strategies:

Talk it through.

When your child has adequate space to think better, let your child inform you what unfolded. New research found that sharing only a story about an anger-inducing incident would make kids and teens become less upset both instantly and a week later. Attempting to explain the chain of events shuts down youngsters and involves their brain's thought portion. Show empathy, so your child is relaxed and noticed.

You should also pose questions that help your child appreciate the experiences of other individuals, and use effective interaction or problem-solving. You may inquire, for example, "What would you do to him?" "How is she going to respond if you do that?" "What should we do to keep this from occurring again?" or "What would you do to make it a little easier right now?"

Responding with kindness and sensitivity to a child's frustration allows it simpler for kids to cope with intense emotions and thought stuff through. By comparison, violent or coercive reactions to the frustration of children lead to the tension of children as they still feel frustrated.

Firstly, consider safety.

They will lash out in violent ways when the children are really upset. Sometimes the first phase of anger reduction is to have children walk out from the scenario and cool down when avoidance was not practical. This, too, will avoid further worsening. Children out of balance require parents to move in smoothly — but firmly — so that they don't damage or ruin stuff.

Reasonable mode of expression.

Children are discovering more from our actions than what we say. When parents react angrily to their own rage, they not only cause more frustration in children, they also demonstrate that when upset, shouting, punching, or being cruel are acceptable forms of acting. Occasionally everybody feels frustrated, so we want to show our kids that you can feel annoyed and treat people with dignity.

Overall, good control of frustration involves children learning to think about and handle the whole cycle of managing feelings, discussing the problem, their internal thoughts and responses, and their actual behaviour and how it influences others or the circumstance.

The punching cushions technique means that frustration is all that requires to be got rid of. That is not so. It is a source of knowledge for ourselves and about our environment. Kids have to learn to understand and cope with this in ways that improve their lives.

3.8 Family Rules That Should Be Implemented By Parents

The thought of making rules of the house or the family sounds like a dictatorship, the very last thing parents want to do for their babies. But when one of those house rules is handled correctly for kids, the effect is order and stability. The members of the family recognize the rule's meaning and purpose. The children feel better, and the tension of everyone (particularly yours) is going down.

Then there is a major difference in any law and the one that is correct. So I requested a number of child educators to recommend parenting laws and house rules that should be followed by parents of children aged 4 to 7. Some are for children, and others are for adults. In fact, most rules are for the parents to obey and take the lead on.

First, one caveat: A list attached to the fridge isn't all-powerful. "Rules alone normally can't get the work done. There must be meaning, justice, and empathy." In other terms, there must be specific guidelines for the children. The enforcer of such laws (i.e., you and your wife) must be simpler than that, and the actions will become automatic. Stick to it, and see progress.

Here, though, there are laws that parents can start following at home.

Use less words

This is not for babies. You want them to communicate. This belongs to you. Since adults speak too much per Kastner — about 80 percent too much. What happens is when they wind up babbling, and a 5-year-old says things like, "I dislike you," sidetracking the discussion and running out of all accountability. This enables us to use fewer phrases.

use of fewer terms also refers to recognition. "Good work" does not imply anything said once. Using it repeatedly thinking, it means even less. The best idea is to reserve rewards for stuff for which kids have battled. "You found how the seat belt works. I'm astounded! "Show the kid you've had his head up and heard it,"

Ask for suggestions if issues occur

Accidents also arise. Instead of saying, "Why are you going to do this? "The correct answer is: 'Oh, look what you have done. What are we doing next? "This stops adults from being continually reactive and thus stressing out babies. "They are just waiting to blow you away. You don't jump in to solve the issue, either. Your child is expected to be innovative and creative according to this law, which isn't a concern. When you are uncomfortable about the strategy, just remember how a child constructs it. They aren't burdened by what doesn't work. Their remedy may not be the best, but they cooperate and address challenges, two talents with long-term advantages. That's what helps this theory come true.

No stop

Two things kids believe: one, that you're still open. Then two: Their basic desires. Sometimes, while you're on the line, these coalesce. Clearly reply, "hold on for a second," then, "thank you very much for waiting," with total honesty. So you just have to finish your paragraph. It might take a while to adhere to this maxim, so it allows regulation over composure and urges. More than that, it teaches them that they are not the sole people in the family with things to do.

Ask permission if it is not Yours

Grabbing is a sport popular among 4- to 7-year-olds. A clear "Can I use your truck? "It's a boundary lesson. But since children are a collection of impulses, they will miss the mark all the time. It's still a good concept because, in the end, it's about consent. You ask before you touch anybody, and you stop when she says stop. "To have heard the sentences is one thing. Having experienced it is something special. Modeling it is necessary, too. A Big Area? Tickling. The unconscious laughing is not a sign of pleasure. When you get going, inquire if they want more. They are having the influence of whether it's going on.

Clear the mess

Children don't want to put stuff back, but by owning everything they've made, they can build up their capacity for anger. It's a law that's fairly simple. Before they quit, if that arises, explain in a gentle voice, "I'm trying to leave it up to you, but if you don't want to do anything, I can't speak to you right now." You 're not giving her any impulse, which is what she needs, but you're offering her a path back to you, which is what she really needs. At first, there will be shouting, but she may ultimately see such strategies never succeed so she may have more control and self-esteem as she finishes a mission.

Do not allow sarcasm

When the company is over, your child goes upstairs. You welcome him with "How good of you to join us," as he comes back down. Cue the buzzer tone. Sarcasm arrives with bark and conceit. "It's never helped anyone feel any easier. You might think you know why your child behaves in a certain way, but there is no way to keep everything in mind at all times. A quick, "You 're fine? "is enough. You are intrigued. You really don't say something. There is an opportunity to talk, and maybe you can get an answer. If this is true, then verify it. If it's not, so you might tell, "It doesn't even fit." However, you 're a man of comprehension.

Give them a chance to reflect

This one is about regulating the urges. If, say, a toy is thrown, instead of the unproductive "What the hell?" reaction. "Actually inquire," Why did you want to do that? "You 're not going to deter or make them feel guilty for their feelings. You just want them to know that they've got options, something that kids don't understand right away. This does not change a 5-year-old, but the idea that there are alternatives is now in effect.

Cool down first

It is an all-embracing law for the house. When people are stressed out, nothing can be argued. You have to remain in charge, so stop for a fraction of a second before you say or do something. Consider it a game for the kids. Play Statues — launch it when you need to use it, and they know how to respond to "Freeze." Injecting humor eliminates stress, and then you can discuss the original problem in a non-reactive manner. The children will see parents who don't get rattled, understand what non-chaos feel like, and be able to carry that forward.

First, Chores, then You Play

It's the world's style. You 're doing the hard stuff, and you have the reward—Coffee, quick ride. Paycheck, work. The main goal is to build individuals that are content and knowledgeable. This implies being different at times.

3.9 Sharing Stuff

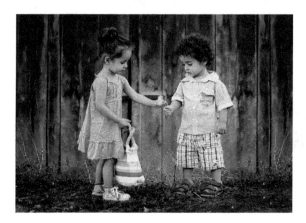

Offer tools. Give words to negotiate and resolve issues with your preschooler ("I want a turn." "I'm not done with this yet"). Sutton has found that he can discourage snatching and hoarding by encouraging her daughters to ask and waiting.

Sometimes "asking" is truly a cry for help from mom, Fraser says. "But Phoebe has become a real dealmaker in her own right after many of those interventions."

• Teach wholesome possession. It is not anticipated that O'Connor 's three-and-a-half-year-old friend, Timothy, would sacrifice Betsey, his favorite stuffed dog. "I am not pushing this one. Similarly, children also need to learn to respect the things of others — to ask even if the owner doesn't use a toy.

• Follow the rules of a play date for toddlers. "You 're going to always need two sets of wings, two feather boas, but seek to promote cooperative play, like turns on the slide.

Meagan is in Lily 's house playing. "Let's Play Barbies. If I may be that girl? "Meagan wonders. "Sure," Lily says. Clark notes that children really start to share well, like Meagan and Lily, as they know that this allows the play more enjoyable. When a kid has great difficulty talking, there may be all kinds of explanations for it. What may help one child learn how to share may deter another. Many kids from larger families, for example, are able to share, while others might protect their belongings. Or perhaps a child was forced to partake too many times.

Children this age, too, have powerful fairness. If pizza is

served up, a 5-year-old would be seeing everyone get a fair slice. Six- and seven-year-olds might be more involved in fairness (Who gets a bigger slice of the pie?). "You 're starting to see benevolence by eight (who doesn't have as much as I do?)," O'Connor explains.

Many explanations why time-out cannot fit right now for you

1. Your child knows that this is an empty menace. You can threaten your child by time out, but don't follow through. Like the boy who wept wolf, threatening to put your baby in time-out and then not doing it or being wishy-washy and only occasionally placing him out in time and backtracking when your child gets annoyed will diminish your effectiveness over time. When your kid does something that calls for punishment, quickly bring him out of time and remain vigilant. (This applies to all strategies for child discipline and not just time-outs.)

2. Your child plays with toys in her room during time-out instead of pondering regarding her behavior. And whether you're encouraging your kid to watch TV or play on their phone or device or laptop, it's not as time-out as it's time to have fun.

3. You are listening to your kid when he is out of time. Why does your kid find the energy and room to worry about his negative conduct and that because you speak to him the whole time, he's out of trouble? Time-out should be exactly that — a break — and not the opportunity to scold your boy, complain about what he did wrong, over-explain why he's in time out, or interact in another manner with him. It should be an opportunity for your kid (and you) to calm down and for your kid to take a break from any conflict or problem that led to bad behavior, redirect his energy and think as to what he should and should not have conducted. It's not a time for parents to chat with kids, yell or express frustration with their child. You can talk calmly about what your child has actually done and what he can do effectively after the time-out is over next time.

4. In time out, your kids feel insecure. If your kid screams and gets mad about being in time out, she's likely to feel insecure. Explain to her in a calming voice that you are only offering her space to be in a peaceful position so that she can settle down and talk about what she was doing wrong. Reassure your kid that you love her, and once the time-out is completed, will talk to her. You may want to sit alongside

with little children (but don't interact with her) while she sits out of time.

5. The time-out will be too lengthy. 15 minutes of time-out is too much for a 5-year-old. As a common guideline, make the time-outs for young kids shorter. Efficiency, not the amount, is what matters: you would like to have your child in a quiet area where he will be able to think regarding what he has done to get himself in a time out and what he can do next time not to end up there again.

6. It's just too amusing. It's not time out if you send your child to her room where she can play happily with her toys or place her next to a TV or give her a laptop or computer to play with. She wants a quiet, distraction-free room to focus on her actions.

7. When you order him to go in a time out, you 're furious, shouting, or both. If you place your kid in time-out, because you're angry, you might give your child the impression that you're punishing him instead of offering him a penalty because of his actions. Just as composure can be contagious, so can be getting angry and upset. It's necessary to convey to your kid that you value him, but you won't tolerate his negative actions to prevent a war of wills and tears and

confusion. Be calm and loving as you tell him that time out is a result of his behavior and that it is a time for quiet thinking so that the next time he makes better choices, not a punishment because you're mad.

8. You give up after having done it a few times. When time out isn't effective (your kid gets upset; you don't see much behavioral improvement; etc.), give it more time. Your child might just need to adapt to the concept of thinking in a calm environment and learn how to calm down. Be consistent and calm, and continue to use time-outs for at least several weeks before throwing into the towel. So when your kid matures, you might want to seek for time again and encourage him and know how to take a bit of a rest and settle down when he gets upset — a very necessary skill to cultivate with school-age children.

9. Time out overuse. Does your kid invest more time in isolation than in productive relationships with you? If your child is in time-out every day, you might want to look at what causes the negative behavior and discover ways to stop the response before it begins. Also, you might want to take into account other ways to discipline your kid, such as taking privileges away. And most significantly, make sure that you and your child establish a healthy relationship, have lots of

meaningful experiences, play and joke and have joy together, and frequently connect (such as holding family meals as much as possible).

10. After the time-out you don't talk it through with your kids. One of the essential aspects of time out is talking to your child after discussing what happened, why a consequence had to occur, and what she could do the next time differently. You teach your child that you absolutely adore her and are there to guide her towards better behavior in the future by connecting with your child after she has had a chance to relax and think during the time-out.

Chapter 4: Grade School (5 to 9 years)

"Big children" are now effectively able to convey their feelings and show self-control, so this is a peak time to set the foundation for future actions. What occurs between the ages of 5 and 10 appears to have a huge effect on what's going to happen in the adolescent years.

Common adherence: "At this point, punishment is just about trying to motivate your kid to do what he's meant to do — clean it up, make it out of the house on time, motivate him to finish the homework on time. "While preschoolers may be tiring that way too, with this age category, it's much tougher as you can't just pull them up and place them in bed or carry them out the hallway."

4.1 Information On Training Your Tween

Take a coaching strategy: Coaches use queries that begin with what and how to help the group achieve its goals. If your son is having a fight with a buddy, ask him, "What difference could you make the next time? "The aim is to help him grow from the errors he committed this time, so that next time he will do better.

Press the rewind button: Give your child a second opportunity where possible. Illustrate what she did wrong, and tell her of the behavior that you would like to see. And thank her when she has it correct.

Use logical implications: otherwise referred to as cause and effect, these should be specifically linked to the behavior of your child. If your eight-year-old is late for school because she was having trouble waking up early, make bedtime sooner the next few nights instead of suspending her rights for television. The greatest implications are those from which the child understands something.

Disciplining your tween

"The tweens continue expanding their wings because they decide to move faster, hang out more, and do more with their friends. This can be frightening for parents who don't want to give up the influence (especially for the first child). The Outcome? A seismic battle for control.

Typical areas of trouble

Backtalk: These are the peak years for backtalk as tweens become independent and would like to see how you react if they assert power. That is often the stage where children want to "fit in" and turn up "smart," so they can imitate the actions of their peers.

Contrariness: Preteens are willing to argue, debate, and take you at every opportunity they get, particularly if they think you're unreasonable. "Generally, problems with preteens are around luxury and independence — how much time they can waste on the internet, whether or not they can use a mobile phone, a later curfew, or can text.

Information on compliance worth pursuing your tween

Don't govern: Involve your young debater in the discussion while establishing guidelines and limitations. Explain your position, listen to his, and then make concessions whenever possible. If your 11-year-old needs to bump up his bedtime to 10 p.m., but you'd rather, for example, go to bed at 9 p.m., tell him that you're going to try at 9:30 p.m., unless he nods off at school. "In the future, a willingness to be flexible and negotiate with your children will win you more cooperative behavior," Carson says.

Negotiate later: Parents frequently attempt to compromise with their tweens as they catch themselves in the midst of a hissy fit, Carson notes. "What we're telling kids is that we're going to be tolerant as long as they argue strongly enough." Stay strict at the time, and bargain later after everyone's cooled down.

Use when and then: "When you've completed your schoolwork, then you can play video games." "This is a term that operates well for this age category because you still give free will to your child.

Have realistic expectations: "I'm not going to tolerate rude behavior," perhaps number one in your catalog. Whenever your tween utilizes a sassy tone (or yells, calls, put-downs or insults), call it right away. "Make it clear you expect respect, and it's unacceptable to tell you to 'chill out' when you talk to her."

4.2 Managing Rule-Breaking

Often children violate laws or don't listen. Even we know that this is just a misunderstanding, as the fun replication of a "no biggie" by my daughter At days, we are convinced that the law violating or refusing to obey misbehavior, or perhaps punitive disobedience.

In these instances, a typical reply is to look for the best restraint-but it is not always clear what is best just that something should be executed. because kids "shouldn't break the rules! "And" Kids ought to know the implications of their acts, "as parents expressed in a session with me recently.

Whatever the reaction, helping kids know, acknowledging accountability, or the importance of listening to our advice is typically the goal. And for that purpose, it's necessary not to use a punitive method. So the child would Not feel anxious, puzzled, and misunderstood at all. They are disengaged from the very individual who should be offering support and direction.

Assistance Rather than penalization

Penalties for breaking the rules can lead to retaliation or withdrawal of a child. So what's that like? It may be an infant who fails to sleep, avoids bedtime, speaks back, or otherwise reacts in ways that attract unwanted attention. Incorrectly we sometimes perpetuate the behaviors of "not listening / not cooperating" pretty much exactly because of how we are attempting to avoid them first. Yet when it comes to kids and learning, two positives are not going to be equal to a good result.

There are magic and sound logic in taking a serene, kind, inquisitive, and comprehensive guide to help children if they break the rules or don't listen to them.

Since an approach to advice unlocks the way for the collaboration. It builds confidence, and it encourages collaboration. It gives children a chance to get to know themselves and others. To add some consideration about their preferences and decisions. It offers you the chance to be viewed as a reliable and trustworthy source of useful knowledge.

The fun copycat moment of my daughter was a strong reminder of just how much expressions actually imprint and affect our children. If we want to support and aid when the stakes are small, so we have a stronger chance when the situation is dire.

These Rules were (not quite ...) made for breaking.

It's critical that we have laws. Especially rules which keep kids safe. It's smart to change rules that match your family beliefs and needs. It's always prudent to realize that your child can check, move, and potentially violate any of those laws.

Testing boundaries is a way to measure liberty, and it is a positive thing, even though it makes one want to stick a fork in our eyes. It's hard, yeah, but having autonomous kids is an essential aspect of that.

It's much better to try to support and direct your kid (rather than penalizing) when the laws crack. As it offers children a basic framework for problem-solving, embracing maturity, and flexing their capabilities of loss and endurance.

Focusing on recognizing failures and misbehavior rather than regulating or punishing, maintains trust, and promotes performance. This also nurtures a competitive group "living for," which you will use from the childhood years and beyond.

Discipline is much most successful because it is about educating, learning, and directing the infant, rather than attempting to make the infant feel bad.

Actions

If your kid breaks a small rule, and it's really just an error or oversight, let them know calmly that it's a "no biggie" moment. Follow up on any incomplete details that they may need not do again.

Check if your child has some thoughts about how to fix her own error. Your child may begin doing this on her own with time.

Notice ineffective behavior? Let your child start again or get a second chance. It might look like, "Can you display a gentle and kind way of petting the dog?

"If you find the conduct of your child is inaccurate and excessive, act gently in order to avoid the behavior. Then follow up with an opportunity for the child to get in contact with you and show themselves. It Could sound like "I'm not going to let you hit your brother! "Step in between two kids. "For you, I am here. Can you please tell me what is happening? "We help kids understand self-regulation and make good choices as they grow when we pay attention to their feelings.

When needed, you can give your child help solving, cleaning, or mending. Instead of "fixing for" mentality, doing "with" helps turn misbehavior into an unassignable opportunity. Your kid will come away with a feeling that she's not only supposed to correct her mistakes, she's still worthy of doing so.

1. Set and hold specific boundaries, so your kid knows what you're actually doing.

2. Speak to your kid with the same courtesy and care you're hoping to hear when she's talking to you, her family, friends, and educators.

3. Try not to give a speech or fixate on the broken rules. Aim to instruct and then step on, assuring your child can continue to obey your direction.

4.3 Managing Lies

Call these ridiculous lies, whoppers or just straight-up outright lies: kids will fib along the way sometimes, no matter what you name them. Whereas a younger boy may make up an intricate story of how a baby sister may not have been hit by him, grown up kids may lie straight forward about completing their class work.

Sometimes also the emergence of revealing lies is abrupt and serious, says Matthew Rouse, Ph.D., a clinical psychologist at the young brain Center. It's a particular trend because they've been relatively truthful a lot of the instances before and are all of an abrupt lying regarding a lot of scenarios. Naturally this needs to be an issue to family members. But if parents can understand why children are dishonest and are willing to tackle the issue, the truth always comes out.

Reasons kids lie

Most parents claim the children try to get something they want, avoid retribution or get out of anything they don't want. There are prominent motivational forces, but there are still a few less clear explanations of why children do not know the facts — or at least the entire thing.

Research new habits

The explanation children cheat is that they have discovered a new concept and are trying to see what tends to end up occurring, much as other forms of behavior. They 're going to say if I cheat on this case, what's going to happen? He asks, "What would he do to me? What will I get out of it? How do I get from it?

Increasing self-esteem and receiving acceptance.

Children who lose faith may be saying extravagant lies to make themselves seem more admirable, unique or creative to pump up their self-esteem and feel nice in the eyes of others. Dr. Rouse recalls the diagnosis of a seventh grader who greatly inflated some 80 per cent of the time: these were very impressive encounters that were not at all beyond the limits of possibly. For starters, the boy would claim he 'd gone to a party, and when he entered the door, everyone began singing for him.

Speak before they understand

Dr. Carol Brady, Ph.D., a professional psychologist and frequent writer for the journal, who deals with numerous ADHD youngsters, says they can lie out of impulsiveness. Once they find it, one of the distinguishing features of the dysfunctional form of ADHD is talk and you're going to see this spreading lies problem multiple times.

Kids will also honestly think they've done something and tell what seems like a fib. Often they would always overlook. I have kids that claim, "To tell you the truth, I figured I 'd finished my schoolwork. I just felt like I had. I didn't think I had to perform an extra task. As that happens, they require guidance use strategies such as checklists, time constraints and coordinators to improve their recall.

And then there are White Lies

And to make it much more complicated, in certain cases, parents that deliberately encourage kids to tell a white lie to spare somebody's feelings. In this case, the white lie, deciding when to say it falls under the social skills umbrella.

Consideration of the lie 's function is critical first. When I do an evaluation, there are questions regarding ways of acceptance that families can check whether the kid is unethical. That's something I should have been digging at for 20 minutes. Which sort of lying, what are the criteria for deceit? The therapeutic approaches depend on the work of lies and the severity of the issue. "There are no clear and fast laws." That means varying effects on various rates.

Stage1: Deception

Dr. Rouse believes it's better to overlook it when it comes to lying searching for publicity, commonly speaking. Rather than confidently suggesting, "It is a lie. I hope you didn't, "he's suggesting a friendly approach where families don't really have an impact, but they may not want to offer it any publicity either.

This is especially valid if the deception emerges from a position of poor self-esteem. "So if they claim, 'I recorded 10 goals in today's football recess, and everybody placed me onto their shoulders, and it was awesome,' and you don't believe that's accurate, so I'd suggest don't ask a lot of follow-up questions.' With certain sorts of low-level claims that don't actually harm anybody yet aren't positive behavior, disregard and redirect.

Stage 2: Lie

When that doesn't work, Dr. Rouse says the parents would be more forthcoming to it by offering a friendly reprimand. "I have encountered cases in which that is an inflated kind of fantastic lie," he notes. "I'm trying to get it branded by adults to term it a tall tale. If the kid tells one of those things, an adult will gently imply, 'Oh, that sounds like a tall story, why don't you seek to convince me again what really happened?' The idea is to idea out the acts to inspire kids to seek again.

Stage 3: Deception

Parents can think of a consequence when something is more intense, such as older kids telling lies about where they were or if they have done their homework. It should be obvious to children that this sort of lie can have consequences, so it won't come out of nowhere. With all the effects, Dr. Rouse suggests it should be something short-lived, not prolonged, and allows the infant an opportunity to adjust to healthy behavior. Some examples: losing her phone for an hour, or finding a work

There always needs to be a portion of conversation, depending on the form, on whether they were telling lies. When a kid has claimed he hasn't had any homework in the week and so the parent figures out he has homework that day, there needs to be a form of punishment for the deception, so he has to sit down and do all the research as well. When he attacks some kid and lies about it, so both the deception and the abuse will be penalized. In this scenario, Dr. Rouse says, you 'd make him compose a letter of apology even to the other boy.

4.4 Sibling Fights

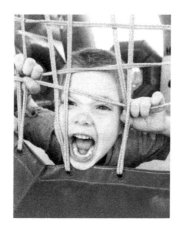

The sibling competition is unavoidable as long as there is more than one kid in the home. The bane of the lives of many parents, sibling rivalry almost always leaves Moms and Dads feeling exhausted and stressed out by all the bickering and bullying, and confused why their children seem to be fighting so much.

They want to find out how to promote a warm and close relationship between their offspring, which will carry forward into the adulthood of their children.

You may connect to some of the following reactions that we have heard from parents about how they feel squabbling about their kids: angry, enraged, powerless, out of power, frustrated, hopeless, powerless, sad, confused, disheartened, frustrated, overwhelmed, agitated and less often amused.

Parents think their kids are going to:

• Damage themselves mentally or physically,

• Have weakened their self-esteem particularly if the conflicts are persistent,

• become bullies

• Never Quit Fighting,

• has bad interactions with parents

• Doesn't show empathy

• Don't think about others.

The various forms of sibling rivalry

Parents are often astonished at the various forms that sibling rivalry can take, and how creative and mean children can be for their sisters. Here are just a few ways the kids can provoke one another:

• Calling each other names

• Blaming

• Stealing things

• poking

• Telling lies

• Defying beliefs

- Having arguments

- Only stare at each other

- tattling

- To break off something that belongs to the other,

- To strike

- Throw something at the other

- Hiding something that matters to each other.

You are probably agonizingly familiar with some of these tactics, and you can certainly come up with a few more ingenious ways that your kids seem to torment each other!

All the fighting seems so unnecessary to most parents, gets on their nerves, and can be upset because they don't like to see their kids hurt each other or be mean to each other. So other parents have applied anxiety as they sound like a smart old owl needs to fix the issues!

Advantages of sibling fighting's

Weary parents sometimes question themselves: Why do children fight? We adults don't believe it makes sense!

In fact, from the perspective of your children, it is fascinating to know about the sibling fighting.

Why Kids Battle

They might be:

• Making sure you pay attention.

• Feels strong.

• Have a break with boredom. Annoying a sister can sound more thrilling than something else that happens.

• Communicate with one another.

• Have direct contact.

• In the eyes of their mother, becoming the 'favored one' by having their sibling seem terrible.

They are all things children desire, but competing with a parent isn't the safest way for them to accomplish such goals; you should encourage them and find solutions and fulfill their desires in a more effective manner.

What kids know through fighting

Moreover, when interacting with their parents, children eventually gain essential life skills.

They may learn to:

• Deal with conflicts for control.

• Dispute prevention and conflicts resolve.

• Be assertive and stick up for them.

• Compromise and strike a deal.

Even for some good outcomes that may result from the battle between siblings, sometimes the almost infinite complexity of the conflict will make a parent wonder: "Why do so many families have more than one kid? "(In particular, 'Why did I have more than one child?')

Usually, parents think their kids would:

• Have devotion

• won't argue

• Be equitable to one another,

• Enjoy one another and want to play together,

• Not even celebrating harming one another,

• Act with compassion and care as disputes arise;

• Don't want to irritate their kin,

• Don't threaten to kill each other if they're left behind.

You may have had some optimistic photos of the partnership with your family before you even got the baby. Such good stuff happens occasionally, and it will melt your heart to see your kids caring and kind to each other.

Yet on other days, you might doubt they'll really get together or even like each other.

You may feel a sense of loss when your expectations don't match the reality as you give up the picture you had of your children being warm and loving to each other all the time.

Even if you may feel sad about this reality, it's best to give up the imagined picture and recognize that conflict and rivalry come with the turf of having more than one child.

By embracing the reality that siblings are going to compete, and there will be moments where they try to do everything they can to harm each other, you won't assume you're going to have to do something bad or do inappropriate for your family.

When you get to grips with this inevitability, you'll be in a better spot to build a strategy to handle the battle.

How your parents coped with sibling competition

Another thing to remember: How you manage disagreements with your own children will be affected by how your parents approach rivalries between you and your siblings. Have you ever noticed some of the following remarks your parents created as you grew up?

"Stop battling now, and I can't take it anymore."

"Don't bother me with your stupid struggles; just work it out yourself."

"I don't know who began it; the two of you should be disciplined."

"Why you both can't be polite to each other?"

"If you're not going to stop fighting, then I'll tell your father/mother."

Often you may catch yourself talking to your kids in the very same way your parents addressed you. This can be because you don't understand why you're doing it, or you don't know how to react.

But when you think actively about which replies, your mom and dad used that were efficient and which were not, you can seek different and better ways of coping with your children's sibling rivalry.

Insights on "images versus reality."

• Recall that, to some extent, sibling rivalry is inevitable.

It doesn't imply something is incorrect with your kids or with the manner you're parenting.

• Children get some advantages from combat.

While it appears to you to be too futile, battling and bickering provide incentives for your children to develop life skills.

• Let go of the notion that you should do away with sibling competition.

If you give up the visions of a perfectly harmonious bond with your babies, you'll be in a better place to handle the arguing and bickering.

• Be mindful of how your parents treated your dispute with your brothers.

It will allow you to eliminate the solutions you now see that were not successful and to be more diligent about utilizing the strategies you see that were efficient.

The conflict between siblings has its roots in different causes. Their behavioral habits vary from one another because they gained those from the individuals they associate with, or the way they respond to others, both within and outside of their house. Society and family have a greater impact on our mindset as we learn, among other things, our values, religious beliefs, behavioral responses. Healthy Relationships of siblings are believed to lead to the positive relationship of people with other people or their social groups. An individual cannot have healthy connections and social activities where there are relationship issues in the family home, hence the nature of home relationships expressed outside of the home.

Relationships between siblings sometimes change as the children grow up. When they begin to interact with the community, human variations emerge. There are turning points where children may experience behavioral change. These arise while one kid is in puberty, and his brother is already in infancy. They have various preferences, and as a result, the adolescent child may think it's boring to interact with younger siblings. They may decrease bonding time with younger ones and take more interest in going out with their age friends. Psychologists clarified that this is because the condition has evolved from the parity between siblings to the independence where the older child would want to try different things, learn further, and experiment, rather than sticking with younger siblings at home. Younger siblings reaching teenage age do not prefer to duplicate their older sibling's lifestyle. They are trying to figure out how to set up their own uniqueness or identity. Growing up, children discover a place of their own where they can share the feeling of connection to someone.

When the kids learned different ideas through interactions outside, they often express the same actions or mindset within their family. When similarities exist with their interests and experiences, cooperation between them is more likely to have taken place. However, a rivalry between the children occurs where there are contrasting beliefs or understandings as applied to their learned principles outside of the family. This results in rivalry among siblings.

In the heat of the moment, you can feel at a loss regarding what you can do to handle the situation when your kids are in the middle of a battle that is really getting under your skin.

If you look at a range of strategies that you can pull from your parenting tool belt in advance, it can help you quickly respond when your kids are fighting with each other.

Sequence of fighting

One of the queries parents have regarding managing sibling rivalry is: "When should I engage, and when is it smarter to allow the children to work out the difference of opinion themselves?"

The following data gives you some guidance on what a suitable position might be to take regarding when and how to take action. We name it the rule, "green light to red light."

With this in mind, as they indulge in combat with their siblings, you should reflect on what your kids need from you. That may help you decide whether to intervene, when, or how.

• Light: green

Standard bickering, with a slight name-calling

The role of the parent-Stay out of it.

• Light: yellow

Borderline, the volume goes up, mischievous name-calling, mild physical Interaction, hazard threats.

The role of the parent-acknowledge anger and reflect the viewpoint of each child.

• Light: orange

Potential hazard, more severe, half play/half-real combat

The role of the parent-Inquire: "Is it real or play? "Interaction is firmly stopped, rules review, and conflict resolution.

• Red light

Dangerous condition, physical or mental harm is going to arise, or has occurred

The role of parent – Stop the children strongly and split them. If a child is hurt, first attend to that child, evaluate the rules, and possibly enforce a result.

What your kids would need at any point

Do they require:

• Love, Respect?

- support from outside to stop the struggle?

- Avoiding getting hurt?

- Time to get an outcome?

- Instructions on dispute management processes?

- Directions to stop tension next time?

- Directions to make revisions?

- Ways to show sympathy?

- Ways to pardon the initiator and to reunite?

Thinking about what your kids might direct you on how to deal with the battle, and how and when to intervene.

Rules

One way to handle your kid's sibling rivalry is to create laws of the family in your household.

Having guidelines in place is a means of communicating the values of your family and forcing you to think about what conduct is important to you and what you want to enforce beforehand. Regulations are an appropriate protective strategy.

Regulations can set a standard and communicate your

requirements on how you'd like your kids to connect to each other in aspects of sibling drama. If kids fight or do not be kind to one another, you can refer back to the "family rule." Include them in conversations on what regulations your family should have as to how individuals should behave with each other.

Here are a few laws that a lot of families find useful to have:

• Managing Controversy and rage

"No hitting, use speech to tell what you are upset regarding."

• beliefs/morals in family

"We respect one another."

• The involvement of parents when conflict arises

"If I get engaged, I'll be determining the result."

• Injury, or harm to properties

"Whoever ended up causing the destruction or hurt has to make amends."

• Ownerships and boundaries

"We will not grab the stuff from anyone else by first requesting."

• Tattling

"No" tattling "to get anyone into trouble; you can" tell "to get someone out of a difficult situation." For instance, a child telling his mother that his sister is just sitting her dirty boots on the sofa is tattling; a young man informing his mother that his young sister is at the edge of the sofa standing and that she's close to falling off is telling.

4.5 Promoting Healthy Relationships

The description below is more common, which supports a parental approach that minimizes conflict. But understand, there will eventually be some disputes, as long as you have more than one kid at home.

Helpful actions

• Foresee plenty of sibling conflict scenes.

It's common for families to have challenges, difficulties, and disagreements.

Do not blame yourself unjustly for the behavior of your children, and do not set unreasonable expectations of family harmony.

What's crucial is that your kids have sound ways of working out the conflicts.

• Treat your kids as the special people they are.

Make every kid feel important. The needs, feelings, and perspectives of each person are crucial.

• Don't do favouritism.

Do not keep comparing your children positively or negatively with each other.

• Remain calm and rational.

Remain out of bickering statements which are just poisonous.

• Make the foundation for actions needful rather than rational.

In reply to the children's common scenario that "it's not fair," tell your kids, "Fair doesn't mean similar; it involves giving what each kid needs."

• Make a list of core rules.

Think about your values for the family. Examples of simple laws include "no bad words" or "no punching." Tell your kids that stuff won't always be handled the way they expect, and even at the same time they may think and feel: "If you're upset with Sara, you should always tell her what you feel without upsetting her."

• Don't go out to accuse or threaten anyone.

Your kids will understand more by working out the issue with each other.

• If you do not know what happened, don't referee a fight.

Instead, concentrate on the wrongful act itself, invoke the already existing family rule which restricts the act.

Remember, by having more children, you don't have to complain about "who started it;" you did!

• Don't venture into lengthy conversations on what occurred.

All that attention you give your kids is a prize for the arguments and fighting.

• Foster interaction and emotional understanding.

Help children create a sense of consideration and compassion for the way they feel about their siblings.

• Educate kids on how to resolve issues.

Let your kids know you think that they can be creative in finding solutions to their brother's and sisters' problems.

• Be conscious of the stages of development.

Young people have difficulty sharing resources. Before they can share, they will "possess."

• Do not force kids to become buddies with their siblings.

This may happen in time, when they're ready, and by their own wishes. You can however, suggest that they treat one another with respect.

• Do not mourn in the presence of kids that they "battle all the time."

They are going to live up to your expectations!

• Don't allow the kids to play one parent against the other.

If you have issues with a parenting choice, talk directly and in private with your co-parent.

• Consider help from outsiders.

If it seems that things are out of hand, you can look for family therapy.

4.6 Hitting A Child Doesn't Help.

Parents need not punish their kids.

The group, which consists of approximately 67,000 doctors, also advised that pediatricians recommend parents against the use of spanking, which is defined as "non-injurious, open-handed strikes with the aim of modifying child behaviour," and said that they should eliminate using non-physical penalties that is embarrassing, frightening or dangerous.

"One of the most precious things we all have is the connection between ourselves and our parents, and it makes complete sense in this loving relationship to eradicate or limit violence and fear.

For example, a 2016 evaluation of various studies found that spanking does not benefit children.

Definitely, you can get a child's attention, but teaching right from wrong this way isn't an effective strategy.

New research has also shown that physical punishment is linked to increased aggressive behavior and will make children more likely to be rebellious in the future. Spanking alone is correlated with comparable effects to those of children suffering physical violence, the latest reports say.

There are possible consequences for the brain as well: A 2009 analysis of 23 young people who had prolonged exposure to extreme physical punishment revealed a decreased amount of grey matter in a region of the prefrontal cortex, which is considered to play a key role in social cognition. Those who were subjected to severe penalties had lower I.Q efficiency, too. That of a group of controls.

Given the limited nature of the research, it can serve to establish a theoretical foundation for certain findings on physical punishment.

And what's the easiest way to have children disciplined? This relies in large part on the child's maturity and personality, experts claim.

Positive teaching involves exercising empathy and "comprehending how to treat your child in various levels of development to instruct them how to chill down when things get intense.

Efficient approaches should both be to encourage good actions, using timeouts, and create a consistent connection between action and effect.

"We can't just take the spanking away. "We must give something to the parents to substitute it with."

The percentage of the people who spank their kids is on the decline. A 2013 poll of 2,286 adults answered online found that 67 percent of people said their children had been spanked, and 33 percent had not. However, in 1995, 80 percent of people said that they had spanked their kids while % said they did not.

There is always a shift in perceptions around spanking. While seven out of 10 adults in the US approved that a "good, tough spanking is often appropriate that punish an infant," as per the 2014 national survey, corporal punishment has become less common over time.

Fitzhugh Dodson said that certain disciplinary problems would be overcome by utilizing his "control wow method."

"It's my pow, accompanied by his wow," he stated, proving how he'd swat the bottom of a child.

I realize some books say family members aren't supposed to spank, but I think it's a mistake. We left a poor woman with no place to go. She gets frustrated at the kid, she's got it with him up to a point, and she's longing to give him a massive smack on the back, but she's been advised she shouldn't. She must, and for her, it's great, as it releases her stress. And definitely, the kid likes it to lengthy parental rants.

So in the 1945 version of "Baby and Child Care," Dr. Benjamin Spock claimed spanking "is less harmful than lengthy rejection, as it cleans the environment between parents and kids." (He changed his opinion in the 1980s, however).

Many physicians are not backing it now.

The latest poll of 1,500 doctors in the US found that 74 percent did not support spanking, and 78 % thought to slap never or rarely enhanced the behavior of children.

This is another case involving policymakers and school officials. Even though corporal punishment is not allowed in 31 states across the country in public schools, there are 19 states, mostly in the South, that either permit the procedure or do not have explicit laws banning it.

In 2000 the academy suggested that all states outlaw physical punishment. And in 2016, a toolkit was released by the Centers for Disease Control and preventative measures to help avoid child abuse and neglect that highlighted the need for regulations to stop physical discipline.

At the state level, though, efforts to do so have crashed.

I believe people look really differently in classroom discipline and parental control.

Even so, the new declaration on the academy may result in a change down the street.

It shows we see the start of a transition away from trusting that it's O.K. Hitting kids in the name of discipline.

Children need to understand that you have, at the core, their long term interests. If the child does not trust the person, then they would never agree to do as they suggest.

Spanking does teach aggressive behavior. I've always stated that hitting a child demonstrates that aggressive behavior is the right way to solve this issue. Is it sensible to spank jimmy if he takes his brother's toy or tries to bite a friend? It really isn't. Parents tend to spank an aggressive child. But findings indicate that children with spanking training are more prone to become more violent.

Spanking is among the most frequently discussed subjects on parenting. While most doctors and parenting experts do not suggest spanking, the great majority of people worldwide confess to spanking their children.

For several parents, spanking can look like the simplest and most efficient way of changing the behavior of a child. And, in the near run, it often works. Studies nevertheless suggest that physical punishment has long-term problems for adolescents.

Here are eight methods to instruct your kid without using corporal discipline, if you're looking for a replacement to spanking.

Put your kid in time out.

Hitting children for misconduct (particularly aggression) gives out a confusing signal. Your child would ask why hitting her is Fine but not Appropriate for her to hit her friend.

Placing a kid in timeout could be a much safer alternative. If managed properly, timeout helps kids how to relax, which is a valuable skill in life.

But in order to be successful on timeout, children need to have lots of meaningful time-in with their guardians. Then, the lack of focus would be unpleasant until they are separated from the scenario, and the frustration may motivate them to act differently in the future.

Take benefits away

Although a spanking hurt for a couple of minutes, it hurts longer to take back a privilege. Take away the television, computer games, his preferred toy, or a fun activity for a day, and he will have a warning not to continue that mistake.

Keep it plain when you enjoy the rights. Twenty-four hours is usually long enough to educate your kid to learn from his error.

So you could say, "You've lost television for the remainder of the day, but tomorrow you can win it back by collecting your toys the very first time I ask."

Ignore mild misconduct

Actually, selective ignoring could be more efficient than

spanking. This does not mean that if your child is doing something harmful or dangerous, you must look the other way. But, behavior that seeks attention can be ignored.

If your kid starts crying or moaning about getting focus, don't give it to him. Turn a blind eye, pretend that you cannot hear him, and don't give an answer.

Then restore your attention to him when he asks nicely or when he is behaving. He can realize, over time, that respectful conduct is the only way to fulfill his needs.

Teach Different Skills

One of the big spanking issues is that it doesn't show the kid how to act properly. Because he was throwing a temper tantrum, spanking your child didn't teach him how to relax the next time he gets upset.

Children benefit from knowing how to solve problems, manage feelings, and make compromises. When parents develop these techniques, it will dramatically mitigate issues with behavior. Using training that is structured to instruct, not to punish.

Provide strong implications

Strong consequences are a good way to help children

struggling with particular behavioral issues. Strong consequences are tied specifically to the misconduct.

For example, if your child isn't eating his dinner, don't let him get a snack in bedtime. Or, if he refuses to collect his trucks, do not let him have fun with them for the remainder of the day.

Linking the result closer to the issue of actions lets children understand that their decisions have clear effects.

Allow Natural Consequences

Inevitable consequences enable the kids to learn out of their own errors. For starters, if your kid decides he won't wear a sweater, allow him to go out and get cold — as far as it's healthy to do.

When you think your kid will gain knowledge from his own mistake, use inevitable consequences. Evaluate the work to make sure there is no real danger your kid will experience.

Honor good works

Rather than hitting a child for misconduct, praise them for positive behavior. For example, if your kid frequently fights with his siblings, create a system of rewards to encourage him to get along with them effectively.

Providing an opportunity to behave will easily transform bad behavior around. Reward systems help children concentrate on what they need to do to gain privileges, instead of emphasizing the bad behavior they should avoid.

Glory be to decent behavior

Prevent behavioral issues by acknowledging your child being good. For example, refer it out when he plays nicely with his family members. Tell, "You're doing such a nice job, sharing toys and taking turns."

If there are many children in the house, give the children who are observing the rules and acting well the most recognition and encouragement. So, as the other child starts to behave, offer him all encouragement and attention.

4.7 Managing Kids Who Backtalk

"I don't want to!"

"I'm not doing that!"

"You can't make me!"

"You're the meanest mommy!"

Familiar sound? You are not alone in this. Backtalk is the top issue that I hear from the hundreds of parents that I've worked with. But is it any less frustrating to know how prevalent Backtalk is? Clearly not!

Backtalk may be irritating and sometimes maddening, but growing up and gaining freedom has a common side-effect.

At all ages, children on an interpersonal basis require a good sense of self - control. They lash out with phrases when they cannot get it because we're ordering them around or doing everything for them.

It's a classic "fight or flight" response – because they're not exactly able to move into their little apartment (flight), they're going to retaliate by checking limits and attempting to get a reaction.

There are several explanations for why children talk back, and it's crucial to get to the heart of the problem and find out which approach would function better.

The easiest way to reduce Backtalk in its path is to give the positive personal power that our children require. We can make them develop by promoting freedom within our boundaries, as well as limiting the Backtalk, arguing, and complaining that nobody appreciates.

Setting the brakes on Backtalk, here are 5 steps:

Don't take on a role

Interaction is a two-way street, and the parents have to "own" their role in the fight for control.

Be aware of your interaction style and reduce the amount of authority with your kids (and spouse) when ordering, correcting, and directing!

The fact is, parents unknowingly add to the power dynamics that so frequently generate Backtalk by bossing children around.

Pause for a moment and swap places with your kids – if you were told what to do the whole day, would you be capable of holding your tongue? I

In the world of work, it's comparable to working for a bossy manager — it's exhausting, annoying, and, most of all, discouraging.

If you spend much of your time requesting, correcting, and guiding your kids, they'll definitely be frustrated too. Rather, invest deliberate time playing, learning, and communicating with them to fend off the Backtalk constructively.

By participating more and ordering less, you'll be surprised at how much more communicative your kids will be, and how the Backtalk will reduce quietly.

Give Attention

Just like the above-described need for authority, your children have an attention bag that needs to be filled daily.

All individuals have a fundamental need for identity and purpose, and when you give your kids full attention, these needs are fulfilled more effectively for kids. Before you say, "Wait! I give them attention, PLENTY! "Let's breakthrough that a little bit further.

I instruct parents to spend 10 minutes for each child every day, as a starting point. We call this "Mind, Body, and Soul Time" here at Positive Parenting Solutions since it has a collective benefit on your kid's mind, body, and soul.

Give power to children

Look for opportunities for your children to take control of their own world - choose their own dress (for a kid) or schedule a family holiday activity (for a teenager).

The reality is, when the need for the authority of children is not met, they will exercise their rights in all kinds of things — waging war at the dinner table, prolonging sleep schedule, refusing to comply in the daily schedule, or talking back.

Children have legitimate authority in each of these scenarios-we cannot Pressure them to consume their vegetables. We cannot Compel them in their bed to sleep. We cannot Force them in the morning to pick up speed. And we have no power over what comes out of their mouths, as much as we desire otherwise.

As a Supportive Parenting coach, I tell parents that constructive discipline is the most successful way to see improvements in children's behaviors. The more positive authority you give them proactively in this case, the less you will have to Respond when they impose their authority in harmful ways.

To meet the 10 minutes basic need for attention of the child and meet the Mind, Body, and Soul Time criteria, it needs to fit the following 3 categories:

It's child-centered: This implies that the kid is making the decisions. By allowing your kids complete authority over how you're going to spend this moment, you're both filling the authority AND focus buckets – looks like a win-win, huh?

Be ready to perform dress-up, re-enact a favorite film, kick a soccer ball around, play their favorite tunes for a dance party, read a precious book, build a Lego fortress – whatever your kid implies for 10 minutes, you are passionately obliged to do.

It's Defined and declared: Give a name for your time together for 10 minutes: "Mommy and josh's Unique Moment" or "Our Together Moment" or whatever name you both come up with. Your kid is able to classify this time together as important and relevant by calling this period together. Naming this period always lends YOU space in the emotional bank of your kid. Although "taking credit" for investing time with your child can sound ridiculous, it is a subtle message to your children that you are regularly engaging in their lives. When you're done, just think, Yeah, I have always appreciated our time together. I can't wait for it to happen again tomorrow!

You'll see a reduction in the Backtalk you are witnessing by investing time upfront.

Spending more time with every one of your kids will dramatically minimize the power conflicts that you experience, and your kids will continue to understand that everybody is on the same side!

It's Uninterrupted: Set aside the mobile, the remote, the schedule, the book — all those items can wait. It is absolutely crucial to give full attention to your kids throughout that time.

If you have more than one kid, find anything the other kiddos can do during this time, so that you can take part individually with each child.

See the Rules

Children depend on order and routine. Although it can sound counter-intuitive, when kids don't know what to do, power conflicts arise more frequently. Backtalk is more frequently than not just pushback against an assumption that has not been explicitly defined or applied.

Although versatility in parenting is often important, continuity and reliability can build you for long-term success. Offer your kids really specific house standards, and set concrete penalties on any child who wants to challenge them.

You don't have to be overly stern or rigid; you just have to comply with the boundaries that you set.

Keep calm.

While your kids put on a Tony award-winning drama show, your role is to be an un-amused attendee.

When you get angry and respond with a "you won't be talking to me that way, young man! "They SCORE a payout for power. Your children can actually talk back and get a reaction out of you – so don't give them the gratification!

Only say, "The way you speak to me, I feel bad. I am going to move away when I hear a certain tone of voice. When you can speak politely to me, we can speak again. "Then, go away.

There's no need for even an alert the next time this happens – just leave the place. You are sending out the signal you refuse to take part in a struggle for power. And when there is nobody for whom to fight, there is no war!

Chapter 5: Managing Teens

One of the teenage parent's most liberating realizations is to recognize what their child is going to do and why. In reality, finding that the same poor attitude that leaves you furious is completely natural, and good for your kid may be quite comforting. That may sound frightening at first, as though there is little cause to believe their actions will change, but that isn't the case. Ultimately, the way they act and the effects of acting like that are also critical to the growth of your kid. This implies training and learning; all in all, the realistic implementation of this understanding is that, in spite of their growth, their conduct is entirely acceptable as is the reaction and any repercussions they should suffer for their poor behavior.

5.1 Understanding The Teen Years

Generally, for parents who fear that their kid's conduct is excessive or felt guilty about punishment, this may be really empowering. Recognizing this fact will also help you to maintain viewpoint when the behavior or attitude of your child gets out of control, as it is purely an important step in their development. Not every child grows the same, naturally, and your child can show some unusual behaviours that may deserve some consideration. Nonetheless, it is very unusual for an individual not to progress with these same growth processes because they have experienced significant delays or deficiencies in growth.

You will brace yourself for those developmental changes as your child is reaching the preteen and initial teen years. This period in your child's life is particularly significant because that is usually when puberty starts. Puberty isn't a pleasant period for everyone. Pubic hair, breast growth, facial hair, shifting accent, beginning menstrual cycle, and so on are taking a tremendous toll both physiologically and mentally on your adolescent. Physically speaking, the son or daughter is passing through a significant developmental process. Therefore their bodies must adapt to these new dynamics and changes. Enhanced hunger, long naps, and prolonged night sleep are all normal occurrences and are only the way the body adapts.

This may be a struggle for all parents and young people to cope with the initiation of menstruation, but the greater difficulty arises if the young girl does not commence her period until her mid-teens. If this occurs, recommend visiting the family practitioner for examination, or taking her to an OB

/ GYN. You'll also want to ensure her habits and lifestyle are safe and not liable for late menstruation. Instead, because your son may not undergo major growth spurts and stays about the same height he was during puberty, a specialist may also test him and decide if there are any questions concerning his hormones.

Both of these bodily improvements produce heightened feelings and enhanced social consciousness. The odds are pretty good that your teen will probably compare the development of their body with that of their mates or other peers. Height, weight, breast size, penis size, and more would be measured and contrasted with blemishes in the face, hair length, fitness, etc. To become very conscious of their physical appearance and to judge their own attractiveness is normal and healthy for your child.

As a parent, by complimenting their many achievements and pointing out distinctive physical attributes, you can help mitigate the strain they place on themselves to appear attractive. Although it's incredibly important to talk about wellness with your kids, it's also absolutely critical that you don't impede their growth of self-confidence. Adolescence is a very difficult time because your child may be hyperconscious with any physical defects they might have; your role as a parent is to help support their mental and psychological well-being, never become part of the issue.

Teenage neurological growth is rivaling the complexity and scale of physical progress. This teenage boy or young woman who just earlier today seemed like a child has suddenly developed into a very severe ball of emotion. Boys in our culture are less inclined to be transparent with their feelings or personal issues when they are frustrated. Alternatively, young women tend to reveal a wider variety of emotions, from anger to anxiety to insecurity, etc. The truth is that all such feelings are felt by both young boys and girls, but culture has conditioned them to express their emotions in various forms, depending on gender. It's important that you understand even whether you witness a kid exhibiting a wide variety of feelings or not, they suffer even though you can't see it. So be compassionate, forgive, and provide your child with the knowledge they need to communicate their feelings. When your kid is dealing with frustration, let them have a healthy outlet so they can unleash their rages like the football pitch or maybe even a bat and their room. Alternatively, build a safe emotional spot for your child to cry or filter other emotions, whether man or woman.

One does not overlook the influence of the powerful "teenage hormones." During this time, both young men and young women experience dramatic changes in their hormones, and their actions will demonstrate it just as much as their bodies do. All boys and girls are apt to switch between emotions of self-confidence (or even ignorance) and crushing self-doubt, both of which may be funny for adults at times but become very serious for certain teenagers. Young girls are more frequently feeling elevated premenstrual signs of mental distress. When you think she might overreact to anything due to her impending time, don't say so. While you might be right, it doesn't alter why she feels her emotions at the given intensity; understanding the source doesn't lessen the stress and pressure.

Unfortunately, it is normal for our teens to live in some sort of hierarchy in our culture, particularly if they enter public or private education (as contrasted to homeschool). High school's social schisms can be as difficult and absolute as India's caste system. Knowing where your child is in the pyramid during this time of their lives should help direct you through a few of their psychosocial development. Be aware of those higher up in the hierarchy that they are more likely to experience increased stress to maintain their social status, and because of their own popularity, they may have issues feeling secure in their friendship. Similarly, those at the top of the 'food chain' in high school can often develop entitlement feelings and think that their social status should be translated into dating, grades, and so on. If your kid is on a lower scale in the system, they might be more prone to deal with self-esteem, isolation, and eventual depression, as an alternative. Teens are often abused or influenced by more popular people who prey on the need to be noticed by the less famous individual.

Never ignore the amount you can assist in contributing your child to become comfortable with the social level they have designated. Too many parents concentrate on having their children climb the status ladder when, in reality, many kids become happier mentally and internally when they are not at the peak. In addition, your attempts to support your child change their acceptance level may do more damage than good to their social status and teach your kids that what others think is more crucial than who they are. Once your child is little, it is normal and safe for you to be extremely protective of their growth. When they step into maturity, it's important for them to know that the environment isn't quite fair, sadly. Most specifically, now is the time to show them that what the universe thinks doesn't matter. Instead of concentrating on success and responses from other peoples, it is better for the mental development of the children to encourage them to describe themselves throughout this time and bear the challenge of their personality and integrity.

One incredibly crucial point to remember regarding the growth of your kid is that whilst its body appears much like an adult's every day, the minds aren't like the adult brains. In reality, our brains typically do not end up growing until our early to mid-20s. It's really common for a mom, caregiver, instructor, or anyone else to start feeling and acting as though the teen would be expected to make choices like the adult. This is also exacerbated by the reality that teens usually feel that they are worthy of making adult choices and so, therefore, advocate for this to happen.

While your teen may well be capable of making a few decisions as if they are an adult, remembering that they are not one is essential to you. Use this information to assist and support them, instead of simply trying to discredit their views. Help them weigh all the choices and all the implications that might occur under each particular situation; in doing so, you enable them to understand how to make adult judgments, even if they may lack any sort of innate capacity to do so. The reality that their brains are not fully formed quite practically often leads to temper tantrums, poor decision-making, a lack of preparation, etc.

The understanding that your teen son or daughter has not done growing up, both mentally and internally, can reassure you when everything else falls. Although that may give you many restless nights, it will also serve as a ray of optimism that one day, when their teenage years are far behind them, their brain will grow completely and they will be cognitively capable of being the person you've always been waiting for them to be.

5.2 Blunders Parents Make

Your child is no longer just a little kid. They are a youngster or a tween — and it's time to modify your parental involvement skills in order to keep up.

Yes, they are perhaps moodier now than they were while they were little. And you've got to think about new ideas, like curfews, wanting to date, new drivers and buddies that make you doubt their choices.

There's no denying about it: your teen or tween is going to test your boundaries and courage. But still, they are your kid. And although they are not going to admit it, they really need your support!

The key is to know which efforts are good enough to justify it, and which can backfire.

Too many books on parenting

Instead of relying on their intuition, many parents turn to external experts for guidance on how to raise teenagers. "Parents may bind themselves into knots, attempting to obey the guidance they read in books.

It is not that books about parenting are bad.

Books are a problem when the parents are using them to override their own natural skills. When the guidelines and their individual style do not suit, parents with their own children wind up more nervous and less optimistic.

Using books to get a glimpse into challenging actions — and then set down the book and assume you've understood what to know. Make sure you and your family know what makes a difference most to you.

Expect the worst

Teenagers are getting a bad rap. Many parents view raising teens as an awful experience, pretending to believe that they can only observe desperately as their beloved children

transform themselves into an unexpected monster.

But this brings you — and your child — together for a lot of sad, unsatisfactory years.

The message we're giving teenagers is that they're just 'good' if they don't do 'bad' things like doing drugs, going around with the wrong group of people, or having sex.

It could become a fictional story that fulfills itself: negative thoughts can actively encourage the behavior that you most despise. A study by Wake Forest University had shown that one year later, teenagers whose mom and dad anticipated them to engage in risky behavior patterns showed higher rates of these behaviors.

Focus on the interests and activities of your child, even if you do not get them. You can open up a new communications channel, reunite with the child you love, and learn new things.

Sweating the Little Stuff

You may not like the haircut of your preteen daughter, or the clothing choices. Or maybe she didn't play the part that she deserves in the play, you know.

But have a look at the facts before you walk in.

Give her the flexibility to make age-appropriate decisions and learn from the repercussions of her choices if it is not placing your child in danger.

"Many mother and father don't want growing up to cause any pain, frustration, or failure. But defending your child from life's truths takes away important learning experiences — before they go out alone.

You 're still going to be there for supervision and comfort, of course — you 're still their parent. Yet encourage yourself to stand back and let them realize that you are there to help them.

Too much Focus, or very little

Any parents, fearing a lack of influence over the actions of their teenagers, clamp down if their child ventures out of control. Others avoid any confrontation for fear of pushing their teens away.

You needn't do all of those tasks. It is about reaching a consensus in conformity and liberty.

If you focus so heavily on discipline, you will be able to get your teen or preteen into line — but at what cost? Teens living in restrictive settings lose out on the ability to improve problem-solving or organizational qualities — so you make the choices for them.

Nevertheless, too little training will not benefit either. Teenagers and tweens require a simple framework and guidelines to abide by when they begin discovering the outside environment.

It is up to you, as their father, to define the fundamental principles of your family and to express them via your words and deeds. That's an authoritarian figure, an attitude that "lets kids build the expertise they need to rule oneself in the best way.

Know, the power reaches further than you might think. Most teenagers claim they want to invest additional time with their parents. Continue to make room for your child during the preteen and teenage years. Even though it doesn't appear, you have a stable foundation where they feel they will still come again.

Ignoring the Amazing Things

If you think your kid is using narcotics or alcohol, don't step out of the way. Even if it's "merely" alcohol or marijuana — or if it warns you of your own youth — you have to act today, before it's a bigger issue.

The years when children are between the ages of 13 and 18 are an important period for mother and father to remain involved. Parents might consider drinking a journey for the teen because they drank at that age. "But now the risks are raised.

Check for unexpected shifts in behavior, personality, school success, and friends of your child. And remember, it's not just illegal drugs that are being abused now — prescription drugs are also in the mix, and even cough syrups and household items.

If you find empty cough syrup packaging in the trash or school bag of your kid, if your kitchen misses containers of drugs, or if you find unknown meds, tubes, cigarettes, or matches, your kid may be abusing drugs.

Seriously take such signals and get interested. Protect all the prescription drugs you have: know what items are in your home, and how many medicines are in each container or bottle.

5.3 Tools To Raise Teenagers

Family gatherings.

Family meetings are conducted periodically at a mutually acceptable period to include a place for a family member to share triumphs, complaints, sibling conflicts, plans, and another subject of concern. Each gets an opportunity to speak; one person speaks without interference at a time; everybody listens, and only good, meaningful input is allowed. Integrate the get-together with rewards such as a post-meeting burger or ice cream, or assign vital roles such as recording secretary or law enforcer, to get resistant teens to join in.

Do not pressure the teenager into self-reliance until he's able.

Each teenager has his own timeline for turning into an individual adult. True liberty requires strong partnerships with everyone, and rebelliousness is never required. Your child's feeling that you are pushing him into autonomy is NOT healthy — that only leads him to become overly reliant on the social circle for approval. If he is not prepared to go to a month's camp to sleep away, then he is not ready. He would be, eventually. Value his schedule.

Show love.

It's a must for teenagers to have careful attention. Spend time telling your teen that you think of him or her. Hear your teen as he or she is thinking and honour the emotions of your child. Do not suppose the teen realizes exactly how much you value him or her.

If your youngster doesn't seem to be engaged in interaction,

try again. Eating things together frequently may be a nice way to communicate. Best still, invite the teenager to get your lunch cooked alongside you. Think to do your own actions in the same room on days where you are having difficulty speaking to your child. Being next to one another will contribute to a discussion beginning.

Know love and loyalty does not equal absolute acceptance. You should control your teenager whilst demonstrating you are not going to withhold your affection based on his actions. When you find out what your teen should do differently, rather than make negative comments regarding your teen, keep the feedback limited to the behaviour.

Make deals, and teach amends to your kids.

If your child has been raised without penalties, he will almost definitely be close to you. Since he doesn't want to destroy the relationship between you, he's not going to lie to you, and he's not typically going to violate the boundaries. If he refuses, ask him if he might render reparations, like restoring the trust.

Keep children healthy and familiarly linked by having computers in your shared room.

It may be challenging for parents to watch electronically what teenagers do since they typically learn more about the machine than we do. Yet work suggests that he would be less likely to waste time on something that you might argue with if the machine is in an open room that you can stroll past and have a peek at what he does. Kids exist digitally these times, but if the internet is at the center of your house, he will always remain close to his father.

What if you brought up your child with penalties, and now she breaks your rules and lies to you?

Helping her learn to accept responsibilities is never too late, but to begin with, she must respect her friendship with you. That implies stopping punishing and start hearing and communicating. You will always have to insist that she consider ways to carry out maintenance. It's a tricky move, as a discipline is likely to make it worse, and she's going to have to pick the maintenance — and yet you also demand that she do it. No, it's not a penalty — it's a means for her anytime she messes up to make it easier, which is something all adults ought to try to do. Even if she wishes to meet you, she can only appreciate it that way, and if you decide to go through therapy and build the bond together, do not wait.

Place realistic expectations

Adolescents prefer to live up to or down to parental

standards, so set strong goals. But rather than concentrating on milestones like having straight A's, encourage your teen to be caring, considerate, compassionate, truthful, and supportive.

When it comes to day-to-day achievements, remember that through success, teens gain confidence, which can organize them for the next task. When your adolescent takes on increasingly challenging assignments, encourage him or her to decide what he or she can do instead of putting the limit for yourself. If your teen gets low, respond with encouragement, and motivate him or her to get back up and start again. Crediting your teen for the initiative is more essential than the end product.

Set guidelines and effects

Discipline is about training, not abusing the teen, or manipulating her. Discuss what conduct is appropriate and inappropriate at home, at school, and everywhere to motivate the teenager to act properly! Create equal and acceptable repercussions for your teen's behaviour. When establishing impacts:

• Don't set Ultimatums. Your teen could view a challenge as an ultimatum.

• Be transparent and strong. Set a clear curfew, instead of asking your teenager not to remain out late. Keep the rules brief and to the point. Allow real implications and respond to decisions or acts taken by your child.

• Clearly explain the rulings. The teen will be more apt to comply with a law when he or she knows its meaning. There could be nothing to fight against because your adolescent understands a barrier is being put for his or her health.

• Be careful. Don't set limits. The teen may not be able to obey. A severely messy teen may have trouble keeping a perfectly clean bedroom straight away.

• Versatility. As your teen shows more responsibility, allow him or her more liberty. When the adolescent develops bad judgment, add further limitations.

Reprimand your child's actions while imposing consequences — not your child. Do not lecture your teen on his or her failures and the hypothetical, far-reaching repercussions that will inspire your teen to admit you were wrong. Do not use a rude, insulting, or irreverent tone. It will cause a feeling of guilt on your child, place him or her in a protective role, and keep him or her from focusing on whatever he or she has actually done. Suggest questioning yourself before you talk, if what you're going to say is real, appropriate, and non-judgmental.

Prioritize Laws

Although it is important to follow the rules regularly when it comes to things like homework patterns and bedtime, you can sometimes allow exceptions. Prioritizing the laws will give yourself and your teenager an incentive to indulge in dialogue and consensus.

Ahead of time, however, ask how much you 're able to stretch. Do not bargain with regard to limits placed on the health of your children, such as drug misuse, sexual misconduct, and dangerous driving. Make sure your teen knows you will not tolerate the use of tobacco, alcohol, or any other drugs.

Set some good example

Teens are discovering how to act by staring at their peers. In general, your acts make more noise than your phrases. Show your adolescent how to treat pressures differently and be strong. Be a positive example, and it's possible your teen would obey your guide.

1. Note that you are a parent, YET a mate.

Teenagers want the comfort of believing their parents support them, they respect them, and they support them no question what — so they want the connection to be a form of affection. Yet they do expect to feel like they've earned some space, and you might also feel a little shut out. When you're able to handle the closeness in an accommodating manner that doesn't take control of the position as a parent to convince your kid what to do, he's more willing to open up and communicate.

Would a close openness erode the respect your teen has for you? No. Do you not honour your friends and emotionally cherish those who really are around for you? If you offer regard, concern, and genuineness to your teen, that is what you will get in return.

And as connected as you like to be with your child, you still need to pull the rank and say no. When you do so often, it is a warning sign of a problem. Yet the teen can also turn on you to establish boundaries they can't create for themselves. Often you are going to have to hold to your principles and say no, whether it's an unmonitored gathering or a really late sleeping. And, of course, your teen would also be willing to use your advice to come up with a win-win approach, which can lead to your concerns.

2. Establish time together, which is secure.

Be certain to check in every day. After dinner or just before bedtime, a few minutes of discussion as you're cleaning up will hold you tuned in and create accessible contact. Also, teens who seem to have overlooked who their parents are all the other 20 hours a day still react well to a goodnight kiss and check-in conversation until they relax in bed. In addition to these brief check-ins, set up a regular weekly schedule with your youngster to do something particularly unique, even if it's just heading out for frozen yogurt or a stroll together.

3. Involved and correct parenting.

Do not encourage revolt by failing to accept that your son or daughter is growing up and that they require more liberty. Yet don't be scared to inquire where your children are headed, who they are headed to be around, and what they will be going to be doing. Get to know the interests of your children and their friends, so that you get to learn their habits.

4. Try to be around after school.

Saturday night isn't the main risk spot for substance usage and sex; on weekdays, it's about 3 and 6 PM. If necessary, schedule flex hours at school. When your child is going to be with peers, make sure parental oversight is in effect, not just an older brother.

5. Stick to the expectations.

The teen will try to be his own self. Our duty and responsibility are to assist our teenagers in doing so. Yet don't ask your kid to accomplish milestones that you set for her; she needs to start charting her own ambitions now, with the help of a parent that loves her exactly as she is and knows she should do anything she likes. Trust the desires and curiosities of your teenager while discovering her special identity.

6. Make consuming meals together a daily priority

As much as possible, Meals are a perfect way to chat about the activities of the days, to relax, connect, and reconnect with each other. They 're always the greatest chance to keep in contact with the lives and struggles of the family and to find brewing issues. Finally, a significant element in the satisfaction and general performance of children is that they know they have time every day to "only hang out and chat" with parents.

7. Hold communications lines running.

If you don't realize what's going on, you lose any possibility of getting an impact on the decision.

8. Foster better self-care

Like nine-and-a-half hours of sleep a night through teenage is required, and a healthy diet.

For early teenagers, caffeine is a terrible choice, since it disrupts the regular sleep habits. Too much time on screen, particularly in the hour before going to bed, decreases the output of melatonin and makes it difficult for children to fall asleep throughout the night.

Stay attached while the teenager goes around the world.

When we have embraced the attachment needs of our child and supported their growth as their own individual entity, they will stay deeply linked with us even as their attention changes to friends, high school, and the emotions that make their soul sing.

Teens may tend to spend more time around their friends than their family when they grow older, but children who are well-rooted in their communities can react well to attempts by parents to remain related. And at each early phase, parents who have appropriately bonded with their kids will stay involved enough in their teenage to remain connected, even if a great deal of effort is required.

Throughout the teen years, it is important for parents to be the mental and moral anchor for their kids. Children may start playing with interpersonal relationships outside the home, but to do so effectively, they will focus on certain intimate relationships staying stable at home. This suggests a 14-year-old who's mainly centered externally is typically searching for anything he didn't get at home.

We ought to encourage our kids to psychologically rely on us before they are psychologically ready to rely on themselves. Too often, we allow teenagers in our culture to transfer their dependence outside the family, with horrible consequences. Teenagers frequently give away a lot of themselves in search of the affection they desire, only to smash into the blunt truth that most teenagers are not ready to provide them developmentally what they need to thrive as autonomous young adults.

5.4 Disordered Behavior Among Teenagers

As teenagers start asserting their freedom and finding their own individuality, many experiences changes in behavior that parents may find strange and unexpected. Your lovely, obedient child, who once was unable to bear segregation from you, will not be seen within 20 meters of you and will greet with a roll of eyes or a door thump everything you say. As painful as it may be for parents to bear, they are a typical teenager's behavior.

On the other side, a depressed teenager shows physical, mental, or academic issues above the usual teen issues. They can perform at-risk behaviors on many occasions, including alcohol, substance use, sex, abuse, missing school, self-harming, burglary, or other illegal activities. And they can exhibit psychiatric signs such as stress, anxiety, and disordered eating. While any repeated negative behavior can be a sign of underlying trouble, it is crucial for parents to understand which behavior patterns are common throughout adolescent development and which may point to more serious issues.

Changing looks

Typical adolescent behavior: Teens need to keep up with the trends. This may involve wearing sexy or praise-seeking garments or hair dyeing. If your teen doesn't want tattoos, stop scrutiny, and reserve the complaints about the bigger problems. Fashions are evolving, and so is your child.

Warning signals for a troubled teen: Shifting appearance may be a warning flag if followed by academic issues or other adverse personality shifts. Also, warning signs are proof of trying to cut and self-harm or rapid weight loss or weight gain.

Added argumentation and defiant behavior

Typical behavior of teenagers: As teenagers begin to gain independence, you will often argue and shout.

A troubled teen's warning signs: frequent escalating of conflicts, physical abuse, leaving classes, falling into problems, and run-ins with the police are also red flag activities that go outside the juvenile rebellion norm.

Mood issues

Typical teenage behavior: Hormones and shifts in growth also indicate the child can suffer mood fluctuations, agitated behavior, and fail to control their emotions.

A troubled teen's danger signs: Rapid changes in behavior, falling test scores, prolonged sadness, anxiety, or difficulty sleeping may indicate depressive episodes, bullying, and other emotional health problems. Seriously take any talk of suicide.

Liquor or drug experimentation

Typical adolescent behavior: At any stage, the bulk of teenagers would pursue liquor and light a cigarette. Others are also seeking marijuana. Speaking to the children about narcotics and alcohol honestly and freely is one way to ensure that it doesn't cause any more development.

Warning signs for a troubled child: When liquor or drug use becomes routine, particularly when it is followed by the school or home issues, it may imply an issue of substance abuse or other fundamental problems.

Children more impacted by peers.

Typical teenage behavior: Friends are becoming absolutely critical to teenagers and can have a great impact on their selection. As a teen reflects more on his friends, that implies they are eventually withdrawing from you. This will leave you feeling wounded, but it does not imply that your teen really may not need your affection.

Red signs of a troubled child: Red flags include a drastic shift in a social circle (especially if the new mates inspire destructive behavior), refusing to abide by sensible rules and expectations, or telling lies to escape the risk of wrong behavior. Likewise, if your teen spends so much time isolated, that may suggest issues as well.

Professional Support

When you recognize the teen's warning flag habits, speak with

a psychiatrist, psychologist, therapist, or other behavioral health providers to help provide adequate care.

However, even when you are looking for experienced help, that doesn't mean your work gets finished — it's just started. As outlined below, there are lots of steps that can be taken at home to support your kid and improve your relationship. And you don't have to wait for a test to have them brought into effect.

Please remember that whatever issues your teenager has, it's not an indication that you've slipped as a parent in any way.

Rather than attempting to apportion responsibility for the case, concentrate on the immediate needs of your child. The very first task is to locate a way of connecting with what they're socially and emotionally encountering.

Tip 1: Communicate with your troubled teenager

It may seem difficult to imagine − given your child's rage or ignorance toward you − but teenagers still yearn for their parents' love, acceptance, and acknowledgment. Positive face-to-face relation is the fastest, most effective way to decrease stress by relaxing the nerves and concentrating. This suggests you 're definitely getting far more control over your teenager than you thought.

To enable the Communication Lines:

Be conscious of your own pain levels. If you're upset, the opportunity to attempt to communicate with your teen isn't now. Delay until you're relaxed and full of strength until you launch a discussion. You'll probably need all the self-discipline and positivity that you can conjure up.

Be present for the teenager. An invitation to talk over coffee with your teenager is likely to be met with a cynical put-down or rude motion, but it's vital to prove you're there for them. Insist on settling down with no Screens, telephones, or other disruptions for dinner time. Look at your teenager while you're thinking, and ask your teenager to look at you. Don't feel disappointed if nothing more than brief grunts or sighs honor your attempts. You may have to spend lots of meals in silence, so when the kid decides to speak up, they realize they'll still have the chance to do so.

Focus on common ground. Wanting to address the looks or clothing of your teen could be a sure-fire way to activate a shouting match, but you can still reach an understanding in some areas. Fathers and sons sometimes communicate with one another through sporting events; moms and daughters through gossip or videos. The aim is not to be the closest buddy of your teenager but to find mutual values that you can explore in peace. If you're talking, your teenager may feel more relaxed opening up to you.

Listen without providing tips or judgment. If your teen talks to you, it is necessary to listen without questioning, insulting, disrupting, condemning, or recommending. Your teen needs to feel noticed and loved by you, so keep your eye contact and concentrate on your kids, even if they don't look at you. If you scan the inbox or read the journal, the teen may believe they do not belong to you.

Assume rejection. Your teenager can sometimes reply with frustration, annoyance, or other horrible comments to your ability to engage. Stay calm and let cool off your teen's space. Try once again later, when all of you are awake. It'll take a lot of effort to connect effectively with your youngster. Don't be scared off; persevere and come will the breakthrough.

Tip 2: Fix Teen Rage and Abuse

If you're a mother or father of an enraged, violent, or abusive teenage boy, you may fear the consequences. Any text message or knock at the door may bring news that your child has either been injured or has injured anyone seriously.

Of course, teenage girls also get angry, but that frustration is generally represented in verbal communication instead of physically. When they're frustrated, young males are much more apt to throw things, smash doors or smash the walls. Others can also channel their anger to you. That can be a deeply troubling and distressing experience for any family member, particularly single moms. But you needn't stay under the fear of abuse. Putting up abuse is as prejudicial to the teenager as it is to you.

5.5 How To Deal With Teenage Anger

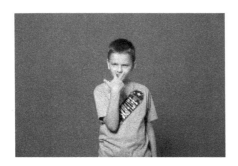

To certain teens, rage may be a daunting emotion because it sometimes hides certain core emotions such as annoyance, humiliation, disappointment, pain, terror, shame, or insecurity. When teenagers are unable to deal with these emotions, they will act out, endangering themselves and others. Many boys in their teens have trouble acknowledging their emotions, let alone demonstrating them, or looking for assistance.

The challenge for the family members is to help your youngster cope more constructively with feelings and come to terms with anger:

Set limits, laws, and implications. At a moment where both you and your teenager are cool, clarify that experiencing rage is not incorrect, but there are inappropriate ways to convey it. For instance, if your teen lashes out, they will bear the risk —

loss of freedoms or even participation of the police. Teenagers, now more than ever, need limits and boundaries.

Seek to find out what is behind the rage. Is your adolescent either lonely or depressed? Do they have emotions of insufficiency, for example, because their friends have stuff they don't have? Does your teenager require only someone without judgment to talk to them?

Be mindful of alarming signs and reasons for frustration. Does your youngster get headaches before they explode with anger or begin to pace? Or does the rage often result from a certain class at school? When teenagers are willing to recognize the red flags that their frustration is about to steam, they will take measures to neutralize the rage before it spirals out of hands.

Support your teenager find safe ways to alleviate their frustration. Exercising is particularly effective: running, cycling, jumping, or squad sports. Also, just finding a stress ball or a cushion will help alleviate anxiety and distress. Dancing to loud, angry music or playing along could also provide relief. Some teenagers often use painting or poetry to convey their frustration in an artistic way.

Provide room for your teenager to escape. If the adolescent gets upset, let them run to a quiet spot to cool down. Do not follow your teen and ask for apologies or justifications while they are still ranting and raving; this will only lengthen or intensify the rage or even cause a violent reaction.

Take action to deal with your own fury. If you always lose your patience, you can't save your child. As painful as it is, no matter how often your kid provokes you, you need to stay cool and controlled. When you or other family members yell, beat, or throw objects at each other, your teen would automatically feel that these are acceptable methods to show their frustration.

Warning signs of acting violently in teenagers

It only takes a look at the media stories to know that violence among teens is a growing issue. Films and Tv shows glorify all sorts of violent acts, many websites encourage extreme beliefs that call for aggressive action, and day after day of playing aggressive video games could indeed desensitize teenagers to the serious repercussions of violent behavior on the world stage. Naturally, not every youngster exposed to violent material will become abusive, but the risks can be tragic for a troubled teenager who is psychologically distressed or suffering from mental health conditions.

Alert signs a teen can become aggressive include:

• Experimenting with some sort of guns

- Playing violent games, viewing violent films or accessing blogs encouraging or glorifying abuse

- Endangering or harassing others

- having fantasies about violent acts he would like to commit

- Being forceful or cruel to animals

Detect signs of teen's depression

Many adolescent disturbed behaviors can be signs of mental illness. Which may involve:

School troubles. Low energy and concentration issues associated with teenage depression can result in decreasing attendance and failing grades.

Running away. Numerous depressed teens run away from home or talk about fleeing, mostly as a plea for help.

Substance addiction and drug abuse. Teenagers may be using alcohol or medications to "self-medicate" their stress.

Self-esteem issues. Depression can activate or deepen feelings of guilt, inability, and social unrest and make teenagers extremely sensitive.

Addiction to smart phones. Young people may go the Internet to flee their issues, but excessive use of smart phones and the

Internet tends to increase isolation feelings and aggravate depression.

Irresponsible actions. Depressed teenagers that participate in activities that are risky or high-risk, such as careless driving, alcohol consumption, or unprotected sex.

Violence. Again. Some teenagers-usually boys-may become violent and aggressive when depressed.

Help add balance to the life of your disturbed teen

Regardless of the exact reason behind your teenager's problems, by allowing them to make healthy lifestyle choices, you can put harmony back into their lives.

Structure construction. Teens may start shouting and arguing with you over-rules and restraint or retaliate against the everyday framework, but that doesn't mean they require them any less. Structure, including daily meals and bedtime, can help a teen feel comfortable and happy. Sitting down together for breakfast and dinner each day may provide a wonderful opportunity to check-in at the start and end of every day with your teen.

Reduce screen time. There seems to be a clear link between violent television shows, movies, online content and computer games, and teenage violent behavior. Even if your teenager is not attracted to violent content, too much computer time will still influence the growth of the brain. Reduce the amount of time your youngster has access to digital devices — and regulate the use of telephones after a certain time in the evening to ensure that your child is getting enough sleep.

Promote workout. Even just a little daily workout will help relieve anxiety, improve vitality and morale, alleviate tension, control sleep habits, and enhance self-esteem for your child. If you're struggling to get your child to do something but play video games, inspire them to play activity-based computer games or "exergames" that are conducted standing up and running around — simulating, for example, spinning, skating, football or tennis. Motivate your teen to try a real sport or find a club or team once workout becomes a habit.

Eat properly. Healthy eating will help to balance the vitality of an adolescent, strengthen their brains, and level out their moods. Act as an example for your teen. Cook more home-made meals, eat more fruits and vegetables, cut back on unhealthy food and soda.

Make sure that your teen's sleeping better. Poor sleep can make a teenager frustrated, moody, anxious, and fatigued and cause weight, memory, focus, decision-making, and disease immunity issues. You may be able to get by on six hours every night and still operate at work, but your youngster needs 8.5 to 10 hours per night of sleep to be mentally strong and emotionally healthy. Promote positive sleep by establishing precise bedtime and removing TVs, computers, and other digital gadgets from the room of your youngster — the glow from these phones inhibits the production of melatonin and boosts the mind rather than relax it. Alternatively, recommend that your teen continue to play music or eBooks at bedtime.

Watch yourself

The stress of coping with any teenager, particularly one that has behavioral issues, will impact your own wellbeing, so it's crucial to take charge of yourself. That means taking care of the body and emotional factors and learning how to deal with stress.

Take time to rest every day and know how to control and de-stress whenever you start feeling stressed. Knowing how to use the senses to alleviate tension easily and performing relaxing methods daily are excellent ways to continue.

Speak it up. When coping with a depressed teen, it's natural to feel exhausted, powerless, angry, or upset. Speaking about how you feel can support neutralize the magnitude, so share your sentiments or find a therapist.

Don't do it alone, particularly when you're a single parent. Seek help from the relatives, peers, school teacher, athletic instructor, church figure, or somebody who has a connection with your teen. Structure and support may also be offered by organizations such as Boys & Girls Clubs and other community programs.

Recognize all other kids. Trying to deal with a troubled adolescent can infuriate the entire family. It can be particularly difficult for other kids, so ensure they are not overlooked. Family members may require their own unique person treatment or medical support to cope with their emotions regarding the case.

This is not going to be around forever.

It's worth mentioning to your adolescent that no matter how much stress or difficulty they 're feeling at the moment, with your love and care, and medical assistance where it's required, the condition will and does improve — for you all. Your teen will surmount puberty issues and grow into a healthy, well-balanced young person.

Addressing your kid's depressive episodes

When children are small, parents are used to dropping in to save them anytime support is needed. When the children grow older, and their issues get more complicated, you have to turn to more of a supportive role, and this may be challenging. This is especially true for teenagers who deal with depression. We need support to get stronger, so we need to seek some help first.

Signs that the kid is depressed:

• Are they depressed or anxious most of the day, for at least two weeks several days in a week?

• Would they really lack confidence in items they used to enjoy?

• Is it modified their feeding or sleep patterns?

• Have they very little power, very little inspiration to do much?

• Will they feel insignificant, uncertain about their prospects or guilty of events, not their fault?

• Did their grades decline, or do they find it hard to concentrate?

• Are they suicidal thoughts? If so, it's important that you promptly get them evaluated by a mental health specialist. When the feelings are very intense, and risks are immediate, you ought to submit them to an ER.

If your youngster shows more than a few of these indications, they may have depressive episodes that justify care. While you can't force them to want to do stronger, there is certain stuff you should do as the parent. And it just starts with being there for each other.

Stay cooperative

One of the most crucial matters that you can do for your youngster is working to strengthen the relationship. Place yourself in their shoes and strive to develop empathy and comprehension. You may be frustrated that a lot of the time they seem away and anxious, and don't seem to do much to assist themselves. But if there isn't something in their life that makes them content or anything that has occurred to them is deeply upsetting, it is reasonable that they may ignore stuff they used to love and return to their space. Depression makes it more difficult to do even the slightest things.

Seek to justify feelings, not dysfunctional behavior. You could say, for starters, "It seems like you've been down really lately. Is this true, then? "Make it clear that you want to try to figure out what disturbs them without trying to solve problems.

Be diligent and caring. Carefully ask them questions regarding their mood without getting angry. Yet parents with the highest motives sometimes fail to understand that their care may be viewed as more important than caring. Do not be dismissive or help to fix their issues, even if you disapprove. Hearing them vent about their issues may seem like you're emphasizing the bad, but in truth, you 're letting them realize you 're listening to them, you 're hearing them, and you're trying to understand — not repair them. People just don't like being fixed. In reality, listening without judgment may make them more likely to see you as a friend and someone they can switch to when they're ready to talk.

Often seek to give them chances to do something without being dismissive of them. Instead of saying, "Honey, you really should be getting up and doing something. Come on, trying to call an old friend? "You might say," To do an errand, I 'm going to the supermarket. If you want to come with me, let me know, and maybe we can have lunch together.'

That may feel passive for some parents as if you're not doing enough. But being present with them is just what they need from you right now, and expressing your approval. It really is a really successful form of improving friendship.

Emphasize the meaningful stuff

Just make sure you note the good stuff your teenager. Going to training, taking down a part-time job, doing the laundry, or picking up their sibling from football practice: these are all positive things they do, and it's essential to encourage them instead of saying, "This is what they should do." We all want to be praised and recognized for doing a successful job even when it's asked of us.

Tell yourself today how many good words did you tell them? How often stuff you said that were negative? How often times have you underlined or attempted to repair their problems? The optimistic will have to surpass the poor. Let them understand you are grateful for them, and they do a great job if you see them taking better care of themselves, completing schoolwork, conversing with the relatives, or performing other things that take hard work. They'll probably appreciate you noticing that.

Likewise, you don't have to say that you're annoyed, for

example, that they don't spend time with friends that much or show any interest in the guitar as they used to. They probably also feel discouraged and should be aware of what will not go great in their lives. They don't want to look like this. If they were able to snap their fingertips and feel better, then they would.

5.6 Helping Depressed Children Get Treatment

If you approach them, some teenagers will decide to go to counseling, and others won't. For those who are reluctant, realize that they may not immediately give up easily to the concept of counseling (or to you), so by opening a door and then waiting quietly for them to step through it, you will help direct them into recovery.

Seek and say, "I know you 're having a rough time, so I have some suggestions of stuff that could improve. When you want to chat about them with me, please let me think. I'm here for you. "Also, it's a good idea to consider them if they have any recommendations for how you could help. You may be amazed to realize what they've got to say.

Be aware your teenager might be telling you to go back. That's fine; it's their way of informing you they need space — although a marginally annoyed one. It is normal for teens to want freedom, and it is important to respect that. You may reply by saying, "I'm going to leave you more room, but if you ever want to chat or hear my advice, realize I'm here for you."

Be prepared if they come to you for aid. Do the investigations. Choose two or three professionals with whom they should meet and advise them to pick the one they are more confident, and I hope it would benefit best. It is vital to find a therapist who is a perfect match, and to make their choice will help them feel a sense of possession over their own therapy, which is absolutely critical for teenagers and sets the tone for effective treatment.

It is also crucial to know that there are many different types of therapy that could be of help to your youngster, along with some well-studied psychosocial interventions. Interpersonal counseling (IPT), cognitive-behavioral therapy (CBT), and dialectical behavioral therapy (DBT) have also been effective with individuals with depression. Be sure your child has undergone a detailed assessment, which provides suggestions for therapy to better direct you.

Many adolescents with depressive symptoms profit from meds, for example, an anti-depressant. While counseling alone may be efficient with mild to moderate depression, a mixture of therapy and medication usually obtains a better effect. If the medicine for depression is a factor to consider, it is strongly advised that you schedule an arrangement for a consultation with a fully qualified child and adolescent therapist (instead of a general practitioner).

Reasons why depression Therapy may not work

If your child is still in care, but it does not improve, question them why they feel so. What is not good with the treatment, or what do they not appreciate about it? Are there aspects they like about therapy? Perhaps you can come together to identify a therapist who is doing more of the stuff they want. If you are contemplating changing therapy, it is necessary to address that with their existing psychiatrist prior to making a choice to shift. The treatment and/or psychological connection may be strengthened several times.

Bear in mind that treatment is usually not effective if the person is not committed to it in the therapy, or is doing so to satisfy someone else. Your kid should try to make himself stronger. Unfortunately, things tend to get much worse even before they seek to support. But the great news is that even if you set the foundations by now improving the bond when they're actually ready, they'll be more inclined to turn to you for help.

You take care of yourself.

Last but not least, it is important to make sure you take care of yourself. Being a parent of one who is suffering from depression can be mentally and psychologically tiring. Know that you're not alone, and get yourself the support. Make sure you allow time for mates and do stuff that you like, and go out. The sentence: joyful mom (or daddy) = healthy baby (read: teen) still applies!

5.7 Guide Regarding Children With Intellectual Disabilities

Steven Spielberg is dyslexic, but as a kid, he didn't realize it. He suffered at school and educationally stalled behind, but realized he could connect on a screen via videos instead of words. His passion for telling tales and capturing the minds and hearts of people via film stemmed, in part, through his dyslexia. He honors the love of his family members as a major element in his success and their assistance of his passions.

Tim Howard has had a great career in the USA World Cup Soccer Series as an expert goalkeeper, and also for the Everton Club in the UK and Manchester United (he played alongside David Beckham). He faced many challenges, having grown up with OCD and Tourette's disorder, but his incredible career was not deterred. Although most kids got bored with sports practice and were going to give up, Howard became an internationally celebrated goalie by taking full advantage of his disorder 's features — such as ultra-focus, huge love, and an unreal ability to follow the ball and not get disturbed by players or fans.

Like other children, all who grow up with a disability (i.e., cognitive, social, or behavioral) have advantages and disadvantages; the two remain together. The problems these kids face and the variations don't nullify the many abilities they have. But concentrating solely on the downsides is common for teachers, physicians, psychiatrists, and others — which often allows kids to concentrate on what appears to be absent or incomplete in them.

If you're a parent to a child like that, I don't have to tell you how maddening it can be. Although designed to be beneficial for treatment, this "diagnosis and deficit" perspective of our medical, psychological, and educational systems can weaken a child's identity.

A strength-based parent-child relationship can be a crucial way to build the identity of your child since it begins with the question, "What's perfect with my child? "Before it starts looking at what could be wrong. This parenting style begins with building abilities and assets before attempting to solve weaknesses. In these interpretations, the term before is essential. Strength-based discipline is not about overlooking or putting a stop to the downsides impractically; it is about where you put your focus first. Before weakness, when you look at the advantages, you will motivate your children to use what they are strong at to conquer what they are not so strong at.

You might not yet know the potential course for your kids. Maybe they're going to grow up to win a world cup or be a renowned film director; maybe they're going down another path. Right now, all you should do is to have your child utilize its abilities in daily circumstances to improve their sense of identity and combat the prevailing impression they associate from them that there is something "bad."

Ways to perceive the resilience of a child

How do you assess your child's strengths? Power is something that offers us an edge, enhances our efficiency, and excites us. Strengths may be unique abilities, such as calculating figures, memorizing information, finding trends in details, playing an instrument, seeing the larger picture, or running quickly. They can also be constructive character traits or strengths of character such as generosity, loyalty, honesty, humor, sweetness, toughness, or bravery.

Strong points come in different shapes and dimensions, and everybody sits inside. When you take a power-based approach with a kid with a disorder, you help them find gold, you know it is there already.

The evidence says three components come together to create power. We ought to hold our focus on all three for the benefit of strength-based parental involvement:

1. Performance (good at something). Look for quick thinking, a consistent trend of achievement, and output that is beyond age standards, or far higher from their other abilities, as your child appears.

2. Energy (thinking positively). Strong points are self-reinforcing: the further we take advantage of them, the more we get. They are filling us with vigor. You will see the amount of energy your kid has while utilizing a weapon.

3. High utilization (selecting to do so). Lastly, glance at what your kid chooses to do in his leisure moments, how often he participates in a specific activity, and how he talks about that exercise.

Part of the fun of parenting focused on intensity is finding indicators of these three factors and giving your child the support and opportunity to discover their strengths. For starters, Steven Spielberg 's mom helped him build home video sets and play with baked beans to construct and film volcanoes that were burning in the backyard.

You don't have to address every hint of strength — that would be overwhelming for either you or your kid. But you will know a great deal about the abilities of your child just by watching what they do and say spontaneously. My 12-year-old daughter Emma for starters is always doodling without really knowing it. She tries to draw personalities while watching television on TV. She sketches pictures in every greeting card she sends to a friend. Seeing this made me discover how I can construct on her toughness by keeping the house filled with art supplies, taking her to art museums, pointing to her street art, and motivating her to enter art competitions.

Study on other positive parental involvement — like using praise, carefulness, physical affection, and engaging with the values and wants of your child — have found that helping kids with autism and ADHD have lesser struggles about behavior, mood, socialization, and hyperactivity.

Strong, practical parenting

By the age of 3 my friend's daughter, Bella, could read the periodic table — we named it her autism's "superpower." Fast forward 17 years, and now she's a satisfying technology majoring undergraduate.

This accomplishment didn't come without the present difficulties having grown up with autism, including the discomfort and uncertainty that she sometimes experienced with social circumstances, especially in her teenage years. But Bella's parents chose the proactive path to having her identify who she was (her excellent memories, her integrity, her kindness, her strong belief in and enthusiasm for science) rather than what many perceived as special about her as a consequence to her condition.

One mother helps her 10-year-old daughter molly take advantage of her strong sense of wonder and love for her friends to appreciate school when she battles to sit still and learn. Mother sandy lets molly turn the talents that come with ADHD into selecting assignments and job subjects that really include her, such as ample resources, imagination, and seeing the larger picture. Sandy starts with the assets of molly first and uses them to effectively manage the ADHD downsides.

It may seem like a lot of effort on the part of sandy — which is accurate to some degree. Still, which aspect of raising isn't much work? From another point of view, the connection between your kids and their strengths makes it easier and more convenient to parent a kid with a disorder. Another mom in my book describes how discovering her son's core strengths, who has Asperger's syndrome, enabled her to better understand him, and how this contributed to making her parenting easier:

Lin has Asperger's syndrome, and it was a shock to me that he has hallmark skill in emotional knowledge. I really didn't believe it until I asked someone else who knows him well. His educators said it made complete sense to them — Fin sees things that some don't and becomes extremely perceptive to the feelings of others, while he does not always react or know what to do about that emotion.

Seeing that this was a strength for Fin helped me understand that he was able to observe the emotions of the people but that he needed help with the appropriate responses. Sometimes when he has a friend over, he will tell me that the friend feels "uncomfortable" and explain what he sees in the face of the friend. Then we're talking, and he can ponder how to help solve the situation. With Fin now that I recognize its capabilities, it's far simpler for me to see and overcome these social problems.

Cassia, Grace, and Fin are all quite verbal. Yet experts have also established recommendations for young people who have learning disabilities who are minimally articulate for utilizing a skills device. Teachers who adopted this method of strength said they discovered different insights about their students, and it allowed them to find forms of making their students know better. Parents will use the app, too.

It doesn't have to be achieved with a device, a survey, or words to bind your kids with their strengths. I have noticed three distinct ways of approaching strengths in the thousands of conversations I've had with parents all over the world. Some parents do this by chats with their children. Other parents connect their children to their strengths through more practical, hands-on ways. Still, others do it by creating opportunities for their children based on strength.

When the kid isn't strongly articulate, either the second or third option should be used. Tune in with the moments that you see your children in action and love what they're doing; pay attention to what's catching their interest. Focus on situations, skills, activities, and relationships where you see high energy, enjoyment, and performance in your child. Put your efforts into allowing opportunities, timetables, equipment, and relationships that enable your child to play to those strengths.

Parenting based on strength is an approach that will help your child see the upsides of life, identity, and disorder. We will start understanding their properties, and step away from identifying themselves dependent on the path to diagnostic deficiency. What's more, because strengths are a journey that the whole family can take, parenting this way has the potential to create wider change and help families achieve happier, more uplifting moments — a goal that all parents are aiming for.

5.8 Strict Punishments

To improve a child's behavior, strict punishments do not work. They are just generating anger, rather. If you penalize your child too cruelly, he will think only of his rage against you and not of the events that transpired.

Severe penalties will just make him think you 're irrational and unfair.

This is sadly among the most commonly practiced traps you can crumble into. Usually, in the heat of battle, when you apply a serious penalty, you 're concerned with winning a fight instead of educating your kid to make better decisions next time.

The attitude of trying to win against your kid, while justifiable, is simply not helpful. That's because you're in the wrong place when you step into the battle. You are the peer of your kid, rather than the figure of parent and power.

Understand, you have already power over your kid, so don't take part in a conflict that does nothing but generates a meaningless struggle for power.

Believe me, I know it's very easy to slide into the brutal trap of punishment. Don't be too tough on yourself after you've had a scene of exhaustion and upset, shouting, "No more mobile for a month! "Simply sound like you're back in charge. It happens to us all. But let's take a rest. The parent-child relationship is difficult.

Example: How long time Grounding Does Not work

Why doesn't the grounding work for the long term? Children typically understand this sort of grounding as "house arrest." In other terms, the instruction to your kid would be something like, "You have to stay home, and you can't speak to buddies."

Yet long-term conditioning doesn't give the kid the message you want him to know. James Lehman, The Complete Transformation ® infant development plan founder, believes grounding simply shows children how to "do time" and does not demonstrate them how to improve their behavior. So, in the end, they do not know the message that you would like them to understand.

Short-term grounding, by contrast, is beneficial when it is used after a problem-solving conversation as a result given to the child. It is an outcome that comes about, regardless of the behavior of your kids. And the child's rational thinking pattern is as follows: "I missed this opportunity and although I should have, I didn't come home. I'm not convinced I will be where I should be, so I've missed the opportunity to go somewhere this weekend.

The trick to a short-term effect is the incentive it offers the kid to want to respond easily again in a manner that doesn't escalate to a result. This does not guarantee that he can make the same decision the next time, so it offers him another opportunity to learn and, if possible, give you another opportunity to implement a result as input.

Recognize that there are ways for your kid to make decisions — good & evil — and receive input from such decisions. That is the best method of educating good outcomes. When you limit your kid to such a degree that you decide all their options for them, they have little ability to know how to judge and make judgments.

Identify the skills she needs to be taught when disciplining your kid.

Nothing like a mystical sentence or penalty that affects behavior. Rather, focus on teaching your kid the learning skills she needs. Reflect on why she originally decided to behave badly. After all, the aim is for the kid to make the right decisions on its own, even if you are not there.

So use repercussions to insist that your child learn the skills she needs to expand her actions. Realize that a penalty offered without that emphasis is just a penalty that will convey little to your kid.

Case: How to manage a kid coming home After curfew

Here's an illustration of how your kid might be treated when she's misbehaving. Let's imagine your daughter is starting to violate curfew, and you want her to remember to get home on time. Here are the moves you 'd be taking to improve her conduct.

Phase 1: Be patient

Don't shout at her, or attempt to beat her at 1 a.m. Upon entering. You are all drained, emotions are strong, and there is little likelihood of fruitful debate. We should wait until morning for this case.

So, please put her to bed quietly and let her know you'll be thinking about this in the morning. Meanwhile, you should take the time to find out just how you want the problem to be treated.

Step 2: Converse

Take a seat together when you are relaxed, and say anything like:

"When you were expected to be on time last night, you didn't make it home. Tell me exactly what happened.

Then let them talk. Then just for a bit, listen. Your child would definitely be making an argument to defend her behavior. She could claim, for example, "My friend who was driving was angry, and she wanted to talk."

Step 3. Challenge the statement

Responding to her excuse:

When your buddy is angry, do you believe this implies violating the law of curfew is okay?

And also pose the same question when questioning the incorrect decisions your child has made:

Next time how can you do it in a different manner?

So you could say, in our example:

When are you supposed to make it home on schedule even though your mate is upset?

Your teenager may respond, I hope next time I'm able to text you and let you know what's happening.

Then, you can reply by saying:

All correct. I would like you to do that every time and I'm going to come over and get you. But the curfew rules may not be breached. And irrespective of that, the duty is to get home on time.

Phase four. Implications

It's time to give your kid an outcome after this chat. James Lehman advises you to choose something related to the misconduct, which will promote her to make better decisions. Have her earn back her lost luxury.

you could tell, for example:

"You weren't home on time last night, and you can't go out this weekend with your friends. So, the limit will be a half-hour sooner over the entire week.

In that week, turn back the curfew of your child by half an hour when she arrives on schedule every night so she will get back her old deadline. This way, the child demonstrates responsible discipline when she wins her rights back.

By the way, due to the severity of the conduct, you will and will change the effects. If the behavior has been very risky, then she will need to be supervised for quite a while, and there should be a prolonged time over which she will regain her privileges. And then another aspect of the effect may be as follows:

"And right after practice, you have to head home. I get to see your computer, and it's going to be held in a public location. You will see friends of yours, but they have to come to visit our place.

And it all relies on the abuse. The aim is that the outcome is related to the action, and the subsequent period is brief enough for the child to begin again early.

Be fair and cautious. With just a few attempts, some kids find it out, and some need some effort to get around.

Challenge the flawed reasoning of your child

Why is this quadrangular phase so important? If you just ground your kid and leave it at that, you are missing the opportunity to challenge the faulty thinking of your teen. And trust me, in the adolescent brain, there is a massive deal of logic that's flawed.

And have them talk to ensure your kid knows what she wants to know. You 're only attempting to shape actions by discipline without fixing the flawed reasoning or giving the kid a new substitution behavior.

You've been too harshly punishing your child — now what?

If you catch yourself in a circumstance where you have imposed an unnecessarily cruel discipline on your kid, don't feel you need to push it through. In anger, decisions are often terrible. Don't step into them.

Know, when you are frustrated, you are modeling your kid's role in how to handle yourself. The kid can understand when you utter something with frustration and can feel that you are in certain situations, being cruel, irrational, or just ludicrous.

You 're their dad. You 're the Lecturer. You may say to your boy, "I was very angry when I proposed that you be grounded for the season. I wanted to treat things very differently. "So continue with the talk on addressing issues. Let her exactly what you expect her to say, and what the current result is.

You are not becoming incoherent when adjusting the effect. Instead, you 're shaping an essential concept for your child — the example that can and should be changed for incorrect decisions.

5.9 Balancing Trust With Expectations

One day, William, seventeen, asked his father if he would be allowed to go to the cinema with some buddies. His dad said no originally, but a couple of hours later, William was informed he would go if he decided to, because it's his choice. William isn't entirely sure it's his call to make. Based on previous observations, if a choice is taken to make his own decision, there is typically a "right" answer that will make his father satisfied and a "false" answer that will annoy him. Sure enough, his dad said he was really disappointed with William 's choice as he wanted to go to the cinema.

If we give our teens the power to make a choice, we've got to be all right with the ultimate decision, even if that's not what we had hoped. Make sure you 're okay with all the options on the table to ensure their decision is acceptable. Restrict their options until you feel comfortable trusting their judgments. If William 's dad wouldn't be all right about his wanting to go to the cinema, maybe he shouldn't have offered him the option to make the decision.

As parents, we all realize that because of their prefrontal cortex, teen's substantive reasoning isn't completely formed. So when it comes to expecting our teens to think through their consequences, we have to practice empathy. We ought to help them incorporate critical reasoning in a decision-making method, which is the idea of balancing the pro's and con's, long-term vs. short-term, self vs. others.

It is in this tradition of matching limits with independence and embracing desires that we are creating a solid base of confidence. Maybe if William and his father sat down and think about the implications of each decision, William would be better able to make decisions that will please his father.

Some of the most important tasks to do as a parent may be having our children overcome adversity. To most parents, as our children encounter obstacles, the normal inclination is to move in "to show them the path" or "to keep them from slipping" If we hurry to assist, stop errors or ease the stress, we deny our child of one of the most important opportunities to learn and value themselves by addressing their issues. We are therefore putting out a notice that we do not believe them.

There will certainly be many ups and downs on the road of parenting, including fresh and unknown situations that we won't know how to discipline. The several challenges we face will make us feel unprepared and daunted. One of the easiest approaches to cope with the difficult parenting seas is to understand how to handle one's own feelings. If you begin to feel insecure and worried regarding your position as a mom, stop to take a deep breath to remember what you feel. You can see a trend start appearing over a period of time managing the emotions. You will then determine whether the pattern is efficient or unhealthy.

Conclusion

People are not born liable, but adults with more intelligence and experience ought to teach kids. Sadly, modern society is one in which many adults and young people exhibit clear disrespect towards each other. Disrespect to kids is so popular, we never doubt it. A young, upwardly developing pair with their stylish haircuts will quickly be recognized. Among them are their 4- or 5-year-old boy, obviously exhausted and annoyed with all the shopping as they move through the shopping center. The mum frequently yanks on the arms of the lagging boy. This is clear that the mother will not hold the needs of the infant to heart. The mom jerks him away when the kid needs to look in a store window. Requests by the interested kid to glance over there are refused or violently resisted. One wonders whether the mother makes use of these pushing and shoving strategies with co-workers in her job. If not, then would why her own child be handled like this? Was it that this child is hers, like some form of property or possession, maybe? The parent stoops down further down the mall so that his face is centimetres from his child's. The parent shakes the kid with a threatening accent. "if you don't quit crying, I'm going to give you everything to freak out for." Father's expression becomes violently twisted.

Does the guy use the tone of voice frequently with his buddies and colleagues? Because if not, why do it for a child of his own? The mindset of the parent is maybe something like this: "It is only a boy — certainly not an individual or a human person." He behaves as though the baby has no emotions or memories. These images, demonstrating cultural devaluation of kids, are popular in Western culture. This neglect is rarely recognized as it's profoundly rooted in our "ethnic neck" that we pull a thousand years behind us.

Adults ought to build conditions that fulfill fundamental development needs for identity, competence, freedom, and compassion to raise responsible and productive children. They identify these "four paths" as the Circle of Courage. There is clear proof that the needs of the Circle of Bravery are based on fundamental ideas, and perhaps even on the human DNA:

1. Relating: The child's need for human attachment is nurtured in confidence partnerships so that the kid can believe in "I am cherished."

2. Mastery: Training to deal with the environment nurtures the child's inborn appetite for information, and the kid can say, "I will excel."

3. Independence: Increased responsibility nurtures the child's free will so the child can believe "I am in charge of my life."

4. Kindness: The essence of the infant is nurtured by empathy for all, such that the infant will say, "I have a life meaning."

In Western society decades, parents sought to raise decent children by teaching them to be compliant. Adults that claim compliance will set very small standards, determined by the level of loyalty. Both children require people surrounding them who are compassionate, supportive, committed, and trustworthy if they are to thrive entirely. We have to become the immediate family of ancestors and parents that once encircled every boy.

References

(COVID-19), C., Health, E., Disease, H., Disease, L., Management, P., & Conditions, S. et al. Parenting Preschoolers: 8 Mistakes Raising 3-5 Year Olds. Retrieved from **https://www.webmd.com/parenting/guide/parenting-preschoolers-mistakes#3**

10 Fun Ways to Help Your Child Gain Better Impulse Control. Retrieved from https://www.verywellfamily.com/ways-to-teach-children-impulse-control-1095035

4 Toddler Testing Behaviors (And How to Cope) - Janet Lansbury. Retrieved from **https://www.janetlansbury.com/2014/07/4-toddler-testing-behaviors-and-how-to-cope/**

A Field Guide to Taming Tantrums in Toddlers. Retrieved from **https://www.nytimes.com/article/temper-tantrum.html**

A Parent's Guide to Surviving the Teen Years (for Parents) - Nemours KidsHealth. Retrieved from https://kidshealth.org/en/parents/adolescence.html

A-Z, T., & Problems, B. Why Kids Lie and What Parents Can Do About It. Retrieved from **https://childmind.org/article/why-kids-lie/**

Brill, A. How To Discipline A Child That Breaks The Rules And Doesn't Listen. Retrieved from **https://www.positiveparentingconnection.net/how-to-discipline-a-child-that-breaks-the-rules-and-doesnt-listen/**

Calechman, S. 9 Rules Parents Should Enforce for a Happier Household. Retrieved from **https://www.fatherly.com/love-money/relationships/parenting-strategies-advice/9-house-rules-to-enforce-actually-productive/**

CPSIA information can be obtained
at www.ICGtesting.com
Printed in the USA
LVHW020505061120
670809LV00002B/187